Secrets of
NATURAL DIET

Secrets of
NATURAL DIET

Dr. Brij Bhushan Goel
D.Ph., NDDY, PGDHHC, Ph.D.

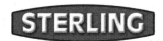

STERLING PAPERBACKS
An imprint of
Sterling Publishers (P) Ltd.
A-59, Okhla Industrial Area, Phase-II,
New Delhi-110020.
Tel: 26387070, 26386209; Fax: 91-11-26383788
E-mail: mail@sterlingpublishers.com
www.sterlingpublishers.com

Secrets of Natural Diet
Copyright © 2013 by Brij Bhushan Goel
ISBN 978 81 207 7996 9
Reprint 2015, 2016

All rights are reserved.
No part of this publication may be reproduced, stored in a retrieval system or transmitted, in any form or by any means, mechanical, photocopying, recording or otherwise, without prior written permission of the author.

Printed in India

Printed and Published by Sterling Publishers Pvt. Ltd.,
New Delhi-110020.

Contents

Preface	ix
Natural Diet	1
Uncooked Food Stuffs (Substances)	2
Benefits of Uncooked Food	3
Wonders of Uncooked Food: A Natural Diet	6
Questions-Answers Relating to Natural Diet	8
Juices	15

    (1) Amla (Emblic myrobalan) Juice, (2) Apple Juice, (3) Bael (Wood-apple) Juice, (4) Banana Stem Juice, (5) Basil Juice, (6) Beetroot Juice, (7) Bottle Gourd (White Gourd) Juice, (8) Cabbage Juice, (9) Carrot Juice, (10) Coconut Water, (11) Cucumber Juice, (12) Fenugreek Leaves Juice, (13) Garlic Juice, (14) Giloe Juice, (15) Ginger Juice, (16) Grape Juice, (17) Lemon Juice, (18) Margosa Leaves Juice, (19) Mint Juice, (20) Orange Juice, (21) Raw Papaya Juice, (22) Pear Juice, (23) Pineapple Juice, (24) Pomegranate Juice, (25) Potato Juice, (26) Radish Juice, (27) Spinach Juice, (28) Sweet Lemon Juice, (29) Tomato Juice, (30) Turnip Juice, (31) Water Melon Juice, (32) Wheat Grass Juice, (33) White Pumpkin Juice.

Various Combination of Juices	29
Fruits	32

    (1) Apple, (2) Banana, (3) Black Berry, (4) Cherry, (5) Custard Apple, (6) Grape, (7) Falsa, (8) Guava, (9) Jujube/Zizyphus, (10) Loquat, (11) Mango, (12) Mulberry, (13) Melon, (14) Orange, (15) Papaya, (16) Peach, (17) Pear, (18) Pineapple, (19) Plum/Prune, (20)

Pomegranate, (21) Rasp Berry, (22) Sapota, (23) Straw Berry, (24) Sweet Lemon, (25) Watermelon.

Vegetables 41
(1) Beetroot, (2) Cabbage, (3) Carrot, (4) Cucumber, (5) Garlic, (6) Onion, (7) Peas, (8) Radish, (9) Tomato, (10) Turnip, (11) Vegetable Marrow.

Leafy Vegetables 44
(1) Bengal Gram Leaves, (2) Broccoli, (3) Celery, (4) Coriander Leaves, (5) Drum Stick Leaves, (6) Fenugreek Leaves, (7) Ipomoea, (8) Lettuce, (9) Mint, (10) Radish Leaves, (11) Spinach, (12) White Goose Poot (Bathua)

Sprouted Food 48

Alfalfa 50

Dry Fruits 51
(1) Almond, (2) Cashewnut, (3) Pistachio Nut, (4) Walnut, (5) Apricot, (6) Fig.

Natural Sweets 53
(1) Dates, (2) Dry Dates, (3) Raisins, (4) Black Raisin.

Honey 55

High Quality Nutrition in Seeds and Nuts 58
Flax Seed, Sesame, Groundnut.

Coconut 60

Soya Bean 61

Milk, Alternatives of Milk (Natural Milk) 62
(1) Groundnut Milk, (2) Sesame Milk, (3) Coconut Milk, (4) Almond Milk, (5) Cashewnut Milk, (6) Watermelon Seed Milk, (7) Soya bean Milk, (8) Sunflower Seed's Milk, (9) Dry Fruits Milk

Curd 67

Various Uncooked Preparations 69
Chutneys, Drinks, Raita, Sprouted Salad, Mixed Salad, Sweets

Food of Special Quality 86
(1) Basil (Tulsi), (2) Margosa (Neem) Leaves, (3) Amla (Emblic myrobalan), (4) Lemon, (5) Triphala

Wheat Bran—Full of Merits	90
Food Combinations	91
Various Tastes	93
Balance of Alkaline and Acidic Foods	94
Calcium Deficiency filled by Uncooked Food	95
White Sugar—Sweet Poison	97
Use of Excessive Salt is Fatal	98
Tea/Coffee—A Sweet Poison	99
Alternatives of Tea and Coffee	99

(1) Basil Tea, (2) Ginger Tea, (3) Mint Tea, (4) Celery-seeds Tea, (5) Wheat Bran Tea, (6) Wheat bran Special Tea, (7) Herbal Tea, (8) Special Herbal Tea.

Spices	101

(1) Aniseed (Saunf), (2) Asafoetida (Heeng), (3) Black Pepper, (4) Cardamom, (5) Cassia/Bay Leaf (Tej Patta), (6) Celery (Caron) seeds (Ajwayan), (7) Chillies, (8) Cinnamon (Dal Chini), (9) Clove, (10) Coriander, (11) Cumin (Zira), (12) Dry-Ginger, (13) Fenugreek seeds, (14) Ginger, (15) Harad, (16) Kalaunji, (17) Mustard Seeds (Rai), (18) Nutmeg (Jaiphal), (19) Piyalseed (Chiraunji), (20) Saffron (Kesar), (21) Salt, (22) Turmeric.

Food Harmful for Health	107
Organic Food	111
Appropriate Food During Summer and Winter	112
Food Classification	114
Types of Food	115
Six Tastes	116
Seven Coloured Food	117
Malnutrition	118
Keeping Fruits and Vegetables Fresh for long periods	120

The Importance of Peels of Fruits and Vegetables	121
Special Tips	123
Importance of Style of Eating	124
Immunity Power	125
Calories	126
Change is also necessary in the kitchen	128
Effects of Non-Vegetarian Food	130
Adulteration in Food Stuff and Detection	131
Poisonous Atmosphere	138
Enhancing Beauty through Fruits, Vegetables and Juices	142
Balanced Diet	150
(1) Protein, (2) Carbohydrate, (3) Fats, (4) Vitamins, (5) Natural Minerals, (6) Fibres, (7) Water	
Antioxidants	180
Phytonutrients	182
Enzymes	186
Lecithin	188
Minerals, Vitamins, Fibre and Energy Found in Different Kinds of Food Items	190

Preface

Food is an important part of health. Knowledge of food is necessary to prevent disease and remain healthy.

Nature has never deprived any animate of food. Man himself on his own started adopting unusual, unsuitable and wrong food and severely punished himself by bringing upon himself thousands of diseases.

Nature has imbibed such goodness in every animate's body and food which enables them to keep themselves healthy and lead a long life. Cows get good protein and calcium for their bodies by merely eating green grass. The elephant maintains his huge and flabby body by merely eating grass and leaves. Similarly for man also, nature has created such fruits, vegetables, dry fruits, etc., through which man can get complete nutritious elements for his health, body and longevity.

The aim of man for having food is not merely to fill the stomach, achieve health or satisfy taste but also for mental and behavioural development. Food has deep relations with our conduct, thought and behaviour. Even today the ancient saying, "As we eat, so will be the state of mind" holds just as true.

A man's interest towards different type of food is believed to depict his behaviour and character. Therefore our aim towards food is to consume those substances which enhance qualities like affection, love, kindness, non-violence and peace for physical, ethical, social and spiritual improvement.

In the manner by which red blood corpuscles die and are replaced by new cells every minute, similarly every cell and tissue of our body is replaced by new ones in approximately six years, whose quality depends on our food. In addition, food must have such substance which enables us to resist diseases and there should not be any hindrance on excretion of waste products, faeces and toxins from the body. There should not be toxic, unhealthy and stimulating elements in food as these elements spoil the mental balance, give birth to impulses and make them aimless and unrestrained.

The medical world has become so advanced that organ-transplant has become a common thing. To find the solution to even the most serious diseases, research centres have been opened. In spite of that, diseases are increasing day by day. What is the reason of the continuous increase in obesity, heart diseases, diabetes, cancer, bone diseases and mental diseases?

There is only one reason–we keep doing new research to treat the diseases. But neither do we implement the ways to prevent it, nor do we try to remove its cause.

If we pay more attention to the prevention of disease rather than finding ways to cure it, then the entire humanity may be healthy and long lived.

In the modern age one gets to see and eat various types of food which do not have any trace of nutritious element. These days the consumption of fried, spicy and unnatural food products is constantly increasing. By this type of food, necessary elements get destroyed and this supports the weakening of the body.

Normally in homes today, chapatis/breads are being roasted on the flame of LPG gas, by which some poisonous chemical element stick to the bread/chapati and are proving to be supporters in destroying our health. Many artificial colours and chemicals are also being added to food products.

Poisonous chemicals and gases are found in abundance in the beverages available in the market. In spite of this, the young generation is constantly attracted towards them.

Boys and girls often feel proud to buy and consume expensive chemical-filled tinned food stuff and tasty canned beverages. The effect of such polluted food is clearly visible on our body and mind.

Preface

In this fatal growth of pollution, stressed lifestyles and adulterated foods, the only way to keep our body healthy and safe, is abundant consumption of uncooked food.

Now considering the subject of taste, the meaning of taste is not stimulation, which is addiction but it means, to get habituated to having food stuff with its natural taste. As bitter gourd is bitter, then the bitter taste itself should be had. If we try to remove its bitterness by adding spices, then it is not taste but distaste.

The main aim of food is–nourishment of the body.

These days, people eat even if they are not hungry and then, to digest the food and to increase appetite, many people use alcohol, tonics and digestive tablets. On the other hand, there are some people who do not have time to eat. They eat food too fast. While eating many people also watch horror scenes on television, giving them distasteful thoughts due to which the digestive juice of glands of our body gets polluted.

We want to remain healthy but unknowingly, we do everything to remain away from good health. We should try to lead a healthy and happy life, as long as we live.

The world's so called greatest medicine specialists and their families, have also become just like the common man and have fallen prey to major diseases and the same situation holds true even today. Several medicinal doctors are bound by diseases in some way or the other. They keep searching for their treatment throughout their lives. The main cause for this is, not giving importance to food science.

The warning of World Health Organisation should not be ignored which says that, if habit of food intake is not improved then in the near future, all the countries of the world will have tremendous increase in the number of cancer and various other chronic disease cases.

To achieve success in physical health, mental health, sexual power and workmanship, man needs balanced and healthy food, which can be possible and successful only through uncooked food.

My wife and I have been on uncooked food since 1986. Through my personal experience and on seeing the effect of uncooked/raw food on incurable patients, I will only say that to fight diseases, uncooked food is the most powerful weapon (Brahma's Astra). To live a healthy and happy life, uncooked food is comparable to ambrosial nectar.

Dr. Brij Bhushan Goel

Natural Diet

The simple meaning of a natural diet is that, according to one's capacity, whatever food usually eaten in cooked form should be taken in uncooked form.

Due to its nature, one can achieve complete physical, mental and spiritual health and not only be protected against disease but can also improve sexual power along with feelings of happiness, strong physical body and spiritual bliss.

On cooking, the natural goodness of food is destroyed and they get converted into poisonous and harmful things. The main cause of disease is eating cooked food. Cooked food takes longer to digest. If the food is fried, then it becomes even more difficult to digest. Many elements get destroyed while cooking and its taste also becomes less. Artificial means (salt, spices, sugar, etc.) are used to complete the taste due to which more food is eaten than needed, becoming the cause of diseases.

Natural food, being complete by assimilate, has the utmost quality of giving good health. Cooked food merely has the unneeded quality of making the body weak. No medicine in the world can take the place of food elements which have been destroyed by being cooked over fire.

What can be a better medicine than food? Just by improving food, all of man's diseases can be cured. Giving medicine without taking care of the diet does not serve any purpose.

Food is the one and only thing, which is capable of keeping us healthy completely. Food itself is medicine.

No matter how deep rooted the habit of eating cooked food has become, but to achieve complete height of good health and get life force, one will have to leave this disease-causing, cooked food one day and adopt a natural diet. Otherwise in reality, diseases will keep increasing and good health will remain a dream.

Uncooked Food Stuffs (Substances)

Juices–Juices of various fruits and vegetables.
Fruits–Various types of fruit.
Vegetables–Various types of vegetables.
Leafy vegetables–Leaves of various vegetables.
Sprouted food–Sprouted grains and pulses.
Dry fruits–Soaked dry fruits
Seeds and nuts–Soaked sesame, groundnut, etc.
Various foods–Milk of coconut, soya bean, groundnut, sesame and honey.

The food for eating, for which fire is required or which cannot be eaten without being cooked, that food is not healthy.

Benefits of Uncooked Food

1. Consumption of uncooked food gives a feeling of happiness in the mind, energy in body and mental bliss, by helping us in achieving physical, mental and spiritual health.
2. It removes toxins accumulated in the body, which is the root cause of all diseases and thus prevents acute, chronic and fatal diseases.
3. Removes insomnia, induces peaceful, deep and relaxing sleep and on getting up in the morning, there is a feeling of relaxation and freshness rather than tiredness.
4. Spreads feelings of being young and vigorous by making arteries, veins and other hard parts soft and flexible.
5. Promotes digestion of food, its proper absorption and excretion which takes place in our body.
6. Brings freshness, promptness, and energy to the nervous system and removes its stiffness, tension, any burning sensation and stimulation.
7. Helps us Increase body weight if it is below average and decrease weight if it is above average.
8. Makes the skin beautiful, glowing, soft, more durable and flexible.
9. Keeps one away from feeling too hot in summers or too cold in winters.
10. It is very important for endocrine glands by helping in the development and proper flow of hormones secreted by them.
11. Pacifies unusually increased sexual urges by inner purification in terms of words, thought and action.

Hence there will be no sinful course by religious persons if they adopt uncooked food.
12. Decreases high BP and increases low BP.
13. Removes acidity created in the body and makes the body more alkaline.
14. Rejuvenates deteriorating life force.
15. Cures mental pain, feelings of disappointment, restlessness and lack of self confidence and it helps us lead a healthy, congenial and happy life.
16. Removes impotency and premature ejaculation by keeping the male glands healthy and active.
17. Removes sterility in women and regulates the menstrual cycle and helps decrease the pain or discomfort.
18. Maintains healthy growth and development of foetus during pregnancy.
19. Helps increase the benefits already there in the mother's milk. The child often grows up very healthy, strong, and intelligent and will have high immunity to diseases.
20. Provides to the body, the best quality pure water mainly found in fruits and vegetables, because of which, we do not require water from outside. When uncooked food looses this water by coming into contact with fire and becomes dry and spicy, then our need for outside water increases which disturbs the digestion.
21. Prevents people from having smelly breath, bad body odour, dirty tongue or foul smelling stool/faeces.
22. Increases capacity to work manifold.
23. Provides balanced, nutritious and adequate food to the body.
24. Provides healthy element chlorophyll (through green leafy vegetables) and fibre to the body. By cooking food, these elements get destroyed.
25. Provides vital elements of food like vitamins, minerals, antioxidants, phytonutrients, enzymes, etc., which are very necessary for health and most of them are destroyed by heating the food.

26. Benefits people working in call centres and other strenuous jobs as they have such long and erratic working hours that most of them fall prey to serious diseases.
27. It is also very important for people doing mental work (scientists, students, etc.) as it prevents lethargy and the mind is seen to work faster and better.
28. It maintains the genes in the body and decreases the risk of cancer.
29. It gives the pleasure of various new tastes, which gets limited (sweet, sour and salty) in cooked food.
30. Strengthens immunity of a person by which he remains safe even from contagious diseases.

Very less food is required for proper functioning of the body. We often have food three times of what is really required. On adopting a natural diet, moderate eating becomes automatic and we cannot eat more even if we want to.

Wonders of Uncooked Food: A Natural Diet

Beneficial in incurable kidney diseases

If there is something that can give strength or capacity to our weak working organs, then it is a natural diet, yoga and exercise. Uncooked food stops the loss of damaged nephrons of the kidney and creates new ones. It takes 3-6 months to see viable results.

Among the diseases of the kidney, the most painful condition is when both the kidneys get damaged and stops functioning totally, and there is no other alternative than to keep the patient on dialysis or transplant a new the kidney.

Many times also, due to excessive damage and old swelling, kidneys reach a stage where they are not able to function properly. In this stage, increased urea and creatinine are found in the blood. This is a temporary condition and such patients start improving after going on a natural diet and also get cured. But such patients are only 10-15 per cent of the total percentage of kidney patients.

Number of dialysis needed can also be reduced in other patients through adopting a natural diet. Those who have gotten a kidney transplant can save the new kidney from being damaged and live a long life, by adopting uncooked food. Moreover, only through a natural diet, can one remain safe from problems arising out of the transplantation of a new kidney. (Cooked food cannot keep the kidney healthy for long).

Increasing damage caused to the kidney, through prolonged diabetes treatment, can be halted by a natural diet. Many patients have been given new hope due to this.

Choosing the right food according to the condition of a disease is important even in a natural diet. Kidney patients have to mainly depend on carbohydrates. One has to have limited fruits, salad and vegetable juice. Intake of nuts and sprouted pulses have to be minimised.

Benefit in Cancer

Those, cancer patients who adopted a natural diet from the beginning itself, for its treatment, are seen to have received a high rate of success, while those who adopted a natural diet in the last stage, as a last resort are seen to have remained free from pain, restlessness and troublesome symptoms in during the last stages.

Benefit possible in AIDS disease

There is just one food to increase immunity and life force, 'Uncooked food'. Hence AIDS patients can also be helped by the adoption of a natural diet. A natural diet offers such benefits which is not possible in any other healing system. Ultimately, a natural diet can be the answer to all problems..

Benefit in other diseases

There is cent per cent benefit of a natural diet for patients of diabetes, blood pressure, asthma, joint pains, stomach, skin and other ordinary diseases.

Benefit in incurable diseases

When there is no hopeful treatment of incurable diseases, a natural diet has often provided amazing, hopeful and cent percent benefits. In some of cases, cent percent benefit depends upon the stage of the disease, condition of the patient, age and patience. The patient is sure to receive such amount of benefit as is his body's capacity to improve and rejuvenate.

Questions-Answers Relating to Natural Diet

Q. 1. Uncooked food is cold. How to consume in winters?

Ans. Uncooked food is neither hot nor cold. Hot or cold is just a matter of habit. Because we have been eating hot food and drinking hot beverages,,uncooked food will appear to be cold initially.

In cold countries, nature produces only such food, which can fight the weather conditions. To fight the cold, fruits and dry fruits are the best foods, which are mostly produced in cold places.

Q. 2. Does excessive eating of fruits lead to chances of having diabetes or it being increased?

Ans. In very serious condition of diabetes, too much fruit cannot be consumed but after controlling the serious condition, all fruits can be eaten in plenty.

The sugar in fruits is easily digestible and is balanced. Sugar of fruits being alkaline and balanced, neither increase sugar in the blood nor exert pressure on digestive glands.

Uncooked green vegetables and sprouted grains are beneficial in diabetes, as these are full of enzyme just like fruits.

Q. 3. Will a natural diet turn out to be very expensive?

Ans. (1) A natural diet appears to be expensive only to those people who have recently started adopting it. Due to being habituated to a heavy diet with inclusion of grains, pulses, milk and sweets, the size of digestive glands and stomach gets enlarged. In such conditions, uncooked food does not give satisfaction, no matter how much is eaten. Till the time the stomach does not shrink to its normal condition, we have to eat more uncooked food than is required. To normalise such enlarged an stomach, the best way is to fast on juices.

(2) While following a natural diet, there will many cheap and reasonable foods which are available in

one's own town or city according to the weather. It is not necessary to eat only expensive fruits and dry fruits.

(3) Those who do not have easy access to fruit, should take 70-75 per cent green vegetables and those with less access to green vegetables should take sprouted grains. Those who do not have access to milk, dry fruits and expensive fruits of high quality, should have soaked groundnut.

(4) Through a natural diet, all the expenses of doctors, medicines and medical tests get removed forever.

(5) Through adoption of a natural diet, there is tremendous activeness and lightness in the body because of which, our capacity to work increases, leading to maximum utilisation of time. Thus we can work more, meaning–more work, more money.

Q. 4. Are mangoes and dates hot?

Ans. Mangoes are grown in summers and dates too are grown in excessively hot Arab countries. They are mistaken to be hot because they are solid foods with carbohydrate. When one consumes these, then the consumption of other grains, pulses should be reduced. Man can easily eat seasonal fruits according to his appetite and capacity, without any problem.

Q. 5. Do fruits and vegetables have worms?

Ans. Have fruits and vegetables after washing them properly. The function of bacteria or virus is to eat the dirt and decompose it. Hence worms are caused due to dirt and rot. Only a person having dangerous rot in his stomach cultivates worms in it. This rot is because of semi-digested grains, pulses, plain flour and sweets. Only raw stuff (uncooked food) can stop the worms from spreading and destroy them. Cooked food does not have the capacity to stop bacteria or worms. The best and surest way of removing worms of the stomach is abundant consumption of uncooked food.

Q. 6. Will raw food (uncooked food) lead to heaviness, pain or gas in the stomach?

Ans. This fear is wrong that uncooked food will lead to heaviness, pain or gas in the stomach. It has been proved through experiments that raw food takes only 3-4 hours to get digested, whereas cooked food take 5-6 hours. Fruits and vegetable juices get digested only in 25-30 minutes and starts getting converted into blood.

Q. 7. Does one feel hungry quickly by having uncooked food?

Ans. The sooner our body gets rid of old habits, cooked food, old dirt, old diseases and starts getting purified, the lesser is its demand for food. We can reach the condition of total strength with consumption of less food.

The more our body gets used to poisonous (dirty, full of poison) cooked food, the more will be its desire to eat.

If one feels hungry quickly, keep taking natural food many times. This state is temporary and will normalise itself after a few days or months.

Q. 8. These days many chemicals are being added to fruits and vegetables. Do they remain fit to be consumed?

Ans. Undoubtedly, the use of chemicals have reduced the goodness of not only fruits and vegetables but all types of food. The only solution is to have one's own chemical free and organically farmed food, or to leave the fruits and vegetables in lukewarm water for half an hour and then use it after scrubbing with a brush and washing them. Those fruits (like apple) which have more chemical sprayed on them should be consumed after peeling.

We cannot escape from the harmful effects of this modern artificial culture of cultivation, but by adopting natural food, we can be safe from serious diseases and remain totally healthy throughout our lives. The body will keep removing the chemicals reaching inside, by way of minor seasonal ailments, such as cold, boils-pimples or diarrhoea. That is why for people taking uncooked food, the problem of chemicals is almost nil. The alkaline element of uncooked food destroys them and hence they are not able to leave too much of their harmful effect on the body.

The goodness of fruits and vegetables has definitely been lessened by chemicals and the resistance capacity has also decreased, but in spite of this, our wonderful body can remain healthy and normal, even through this lessened quality food.

Cooked fruits and vegetables cannot retaliate against even one per cent of such chemicals. Only natural living food can best retaliate against these chemicals. Hence we should freely eat natural food available in whichever way and enjoy it. If 100 per cent health is not possible, even 80 percent is enough as at least we will not be sick.

The most harmful effect of chemicals is on grains, pulses, milk and non-vegetarian food. All these are very acidic, and acids of chemical make them doubly harmful.

Sprouted grains are best solution to be safe from the ill effects of chemicals. On being sprouted, the chemicals in them become weak.

Wash the green leafy vegetables properly in running water and use them.

The dry fruits in which sulphur is mixed should not be eaten.

Q. 9. On being on a natural diet, does body weight decrease too much and one starts looking too thin?

Ans. All the animates of this world keep their normal body weight. This is not merely due to food but all or most of them do hard labour and running around and use their body muscles a lot. The better the use of muscles, the more are the number of new cells produced in that part. This is the reason why they appear to be masters of powerful, strong, active, beautiful and toned bodies.

For the one who stays on a natural diet but does not do light exercise, yogasana or walking and does not use muscles properly, the muscles of such a person, in absence or limitation of use, will remain in contracted form and there will be no improvement in their shape. In such a condition, the weight of such a person remains less and there is limited fat on the body.

People whose body-built is lean and thin, will have to take the help of heavy muscular exercises or hard labour to keep their weight normal and balanced. These people cannot increase their weight by only yogasana or morning walk. They will have to take help of those exercises which involve good use of muscles.

Those who adopt a natural diet start losing body weight for the first few months, which was accumulated due to dirt, weak cells and cooked food. After a limit, decrease in weight stops automatically. This weight loss process may continue for six months to one year, because a natural diet does not tolerate even a single dirt, unaltered weak cell or unhealthy fats.

A normal person may appear as thin and sick, but this incident happens more with one who is seriously laden with dirt or illness.

This is a temporary state, a state which eradicates all the old and takes the person towards the new. Initially, many ups and downs are experienced in this stage. Alternate periods of activeness and weakness and some other symptoms continue to be experienced.

Then suddenly a change comes and all these ups and downs, symptoms and weaknesses automatically end and the stage starts moving in the opposite direction. The lost weight start coming back on its own, new cells are made and the whole body does new production only. The skin starts to glow, refreshed and the body returns to its natural built.

It is nature's simple rule- first waste excretion, and then new production. The more the body remains free of dirt and disease, the sooner will it reflect the wonderful benefits of a natural diet.

Q.10. Is it necessary to completely remain on a natural diet? Is there any harm in taking cooked food along with it?

Ans. Remaining totally on uncooked food depends upon situations, atmosphere, habits and availability of things. It depends upon your thoughts and strong willpower.

A natural diet is definitely the call of nature and order and is ideally a complete diet. The dryness and harmful effect of cooked food can be known by remaining on a natural diet for a few months.

If the cooked food is simple, then it can be easily taken regularly in small quantities, but the one which is heavier should be consumed once in a while. If such food is not consumed too much at a time but in small quantities, then there is no possibility of harm.

Cooked food has one problem- due to old habit, tradition, taste, its quantity goes on increasing and the quantity of uncooked food starts decreasing even without our realisation. Many times after eating enough cooked food, we take one or two raw carrots and think that we are making good use of uncooked food. In an entire day, by eating one or two fruits or drinking juice, we think we are taking more uncooked food but this is only a misconception. Therefore one should make such routine in which the body does get its required quantity of uncooked food in the entire day.

Note-In incurable diseases, following a natural diet is necessary because consumption of even a little cooked food can weaken the pace of health improvement.

Juices

The juices taken out of fruits and vegetables contain great nutritious and medicinal elements. They also contain various types of important minerals, vitamins, antioxidants, enzymes and phytonutrients. Therefore, juices provide many required elements to the body and purify the blood. It dissolves and removes the toxins accumulated in the body and provides the necessary elements for production of new cells. Therefore, juices are useful in every disease, by themselves or in combination with other foods. In fatal diseases such as cancer, juices are specially beneficial. It improves immunity and helps in proper functioning of endocrine glands of our body.

For people with weak digestion, juices of various fruits and vegetables are very beneficial.

To obtain necessary elements, consumption of fruits and vegetables in large amount cannot be done alone but its juices can be had in that quantity. Necessary elements in juices quickly reach various parts of the body through blood and therefore benefit faster.

To get relief from heat, if we consume juices instead of having various types of cold drinks from the market, then it give great benefits. By changing the types of juice consumed, we can enjoy different tastes. For beauty and health, juices should be consumed every day. It is very necessary for children and pregnant women.

Consumption of juices is an excellent treatment for removing the addiction to intoxicating drugs.

Precautions

1. Always drink fresh juice; do not drink juice kept for a long time.

2. Drink the juice slowly.
3. Never heat the juice.
4. Never add salt or sugar to juice.
5. Take fruit juices and vegetable juices separately.
6. Before extracting juice, wash the leaves, vegetables and fruits properly.
7. Take juices and solid food at different times.

Note–Due to preservatives, consumption of tinned juices is very harmful.

Various Juices

1. *Amla (Emblic myrobalan) Juice*

Amla is available from November to March.

Grate two fresh and big amlas, mix its juice with a little honey and take it every morning with a cup of milk. Within a few days, you will experience new strength and activeness in your body.

Amla is the best source of vitamin C, which is necessary for sensory nerves, liver, gall bladder and proper functioning of the blood.

It purifies the blood and improves immunity. Amla strengthens the heart, hair and various glands and maintains strength during old age. It has calcium and iron in abundance and is useful in prevention of anaemia and imbalanced blood flow. By consuming amla juice daily, anaemia, acidity, indigestion, nervous and urinary related diseases can be prevented. Those who want continued health and youthfulness should definitely take the juice of two amlas daily.

Amla juice improves eyesight. It is beneficial in gout and jaundice and gives relief in bone disease and ulcer. Regular consumption of amla juice makes the hair, long, thick and black and keeps the skin healthy and free from disease.

2. Apple Juice

Vitamins A and B, minerals, iron and calcium are found in this. This also has potassium in abundance which is helpful in gout. It benefits people having acidity and destroys the germs in the stomach and intestines. It is especially beneficial in anaemia and improves appetite. Apple juice is helpful in the kidneys clean and prevents the formation of stones. It is also helpful in treating gas and diarrhoea.

If the child is not able to digest milk, then giving apple juice between short intervals help. It has a phytonutrient named Phenolic Compound which prevents heart disease.

Its juice should be consumed immediately. If mixed with honey, it works like a tonic.

3. Bael (Wood-apple) Juice

Soak the pulp of a bael in water for 1-2 hour, mash it properly and then strain it. Add desired water to it. If you wish, you can add honey too. Drinking this juice leads to cleansing of the stomach. Constipation is removed and foul smelling gas is discharged. It stops diarrhoea, swelling of intestines and piles and improves the working capacity of intestines. Appetite is improved and sunstroke are prevented in summers. It also helps in treating ulcer.

4. Banana Stem Juice

This is beneficial in kidney and liver diseases and stops the formation of kidney stones. It reduces the amount of cholesterol in blood. T.B. patients should definitely consume its juice every day. It removes poisonous substances from the body and therefore, is beneficial in every disease.

5. Basil Juice

Consuming basil juice mixed with water on an empty stomach every day, improves body strength and memory power.

It improves digestive power of the stomach; is a worm-destroyer. Basil juice stops vomiting immediately. It is very helpful in malaria. It improves the working capacity of the kidneys and is very beneficial in treating acidity, constipation, white spots and obesity. It is very beneficial when given in 3-3 grams to patients of fever, cough and asthma. Patients with internal stones should be given basil juice mixed with honey for 6 months.

Cough, cold, fever, diarrhoea, vomiting problems, etc of children can be cured by basil juice. It reduces blood cholesterol level improves immunity and infectious diseases are prevented.

6. Beetroot Juice

Sodium and potassium are found in this. By adding 1 teaspoon lemon juice to beetroot juice, its medicinal qualities are improved, which is useful in jaundice, vomiting and nausea. This juice is most beneficial in anaemia, general weakness and nervous weakness. When consumed along with carrot juice, it cleans the blood. It breaks down kidney stones. It strengthens the nails and improves memory power. Beetroot juice mixed with lemon and honey helps in bringing down swelling of the liver. Mixing of turmeric to beetroot and carrot juice and consuming it, lightens the complexion. By taking a mixture of beetroot and carrot juice, kidneys are cleaned and it is especially helpful in female diseases. (It is better to take more of carrot juice and less of beetroot juice in such cases). It has a phytonutrient called Betanin, which prevents heart disease and cancer.

7. Bottle Gourd (White Gourd) Juice

Bottle Gourd juice is full of medicinal value. Being rich in potassium, it is beneficial, normally for all diseases. Its juice helps considerably in treating jaundice. For heart and diabetic patients it is comparable to immortal nectar. It is beneficial in gout, acidity, ulcer and high BP diseases. It gives strength to the brain and regulates digestion. It helps in treating urinary diseases. On regular consumption of one glass of its juice, with 7 basil leaves and 7 mint leaves and little ginger mixed to it, obesity is reduced.

8. Cabbage Juice

Cabbage juice is the most effective treatment for ulcer and constipation. Calcium, phosphorus, potassium, chlorine and sodium are present in abundance in cabbage. All these alkali clean the blood and the body. Cabbage juice is especially beneficial in joint pain, blood disorders, bone pains, nervous weakness, weakness of the eyes, skin diseases as well as nails and hair problems. Cabbage and carrot juice when taken in equal proportion, prevents formation of gas.

Gives strength to the brain and keeps the muscles healthy. It is especially beneficial in treating unnatural bleeding, piles, obesity and high BP. Many types of phytonutrients are found in this which prevents cancer.

9. Carrot Juice

Carrot juice has Vitamin A in abundance and it gets digested easily. It also has vitamins B, C, D, E and K. Drinking carrot juice increases appetite and strengthens the digestive system. Carrot juice strengthens the teeth also. It protects the nervous system. It has elements such as sodium, potassium, calcium, magnesium and iron. Pregnant ladies need not take calcium supplements, if they consume carrot juice. It is beneficial in treating eye weakness, ulcer and cancer. Carrot juice has elements to increase immunity and strengthen weak cells. Carrot juice gives immediate relief in acidity. Carrot juice has been proved to be effective in repairing internal damage caused due to prolonged illness. Bleeding from the gum stops and bad breath is also removed by it.

Regular consumption of carrot juice removes dryness of the skin. Its consumption reduces the possibility of breast cancer in women. Helps treats sterility and improves virility of men. Regular consumption of carrot juice makes the skin glow. Giving 2-3 spoons of carrot juice daily to weak children makes them healthy and strong. Daily consumption of carrot juice by breast feeding mothers also increases milk production.

Carrot and spinach juice when taken in equal proportion, gives benefits in diabetes. Its juice is very beneficial in treating gout, leucorrhoea, tuberculosis, liver problem, piles and kidney disease. It is also very helpful in treating gall bladder and kidney stone problems.

Asthma patients should definitely consume carrot juice. It is very beneficial in treating the swelling of the large intestine if taken along with beetroot and cucumber juice.

It has a phytonutrient named Beta-Carotene which stops cancer. It keeps ageing away and stops the harmful effects of diabetes.

10. Coconut Water

Coconut water is a naturally sterilized, mineral water. It destroys the poisonous effect of medicines. It is a tasty beverage, which is also helpful in digestion. It is completely safe for the children and becomes an effective tonic when taken after mixing honey to it.

Coconut water is very effective in cholera. It removes the poisonous germs of cholera from the intestines. If somebody feels dehydrated, then he should be given coconut water mixed with lemon juice.

It pacifies burning feeling in the stomach. Coconut water has sufficient chlorine and potassium. It is especially beneficial in treating kidney diseases, low urination, stone, toxaemia of pregnancy, excessive albumin, measles and typhoid.

When there is vomiting or nausea in children and pregnant women, coconut water mixed with lemon juice is beneficial.

Coconut water is very useful in treating all types of contagious diseases as well as asthma and ulcers. Those who have nettle rash (skin allergy) must take coconut water.

If pregnant women consume the water of one coconut daily, then the child born will be physically beautiful.

11. Cucumber Juice

Cucumber juice has potassium in abundance. It balances the acid and alkali elements in the body. It is beneficial in treating stomach ulcer, acidity and constipation. Combined juice of cucumber, carrot and beetroot, lowers the level of uric acid. It is especially beneficial in removing the feeling of burning sensation while urinating. Combined juice of cucumber, carrot and spinach, improves growth of hair. It is beneficial in treating diabetes and skin diseases. It has vitamins A, B, C and many other minerals. It is very good for the skin and is helpful in treating allergy.

12. Fenugreek Leaves Juice

Fenugreek is the second most popular leafy vegetable in use throughout India. Vitamin B, calcium, phosphorous and iron, are found in this. Juice of fenugreek leaves acts like medicine in treating cirrhosis of liver, tuberculosis, jaundice, bile and heart related diseases. If one teaspoon of fenugreek leaves juice is taken every day in the morning, then diabetes can be controlled at the initial stage.

13. Garlic Juice

Garlic juice is a good blood purifier. It removes uric acid and is useful in treating high BP, arthritis, mental conditions, cough and in intestinal problems. Kills the germs of the stomach and strengthen the male reproductive organs. Removes indigestion and is beneficial in gout. Apart from these, it is beneficial in treating paralysis, heart diseases, cold and incurable diseases of the stomach. Its juice should be mixed in water for consumption.

14. Giloe Juice

Giloe plant is a creeper, which grows very fast and its juice is pungent and bitter and is highly beneficial. Giloe juice increases digestive powers and is destroyer of vatta, pitta and cough. This juice improves immunity. All types of fever, acidity, bile, anaemia, bowels with flatulence and nervous weakness, etc., can be cured by it.

15. Ginger Juice

This is destroys worms, removes stomach pain and keeps the digestive system healthy. It is very useful in treating asthma, cold and cough and reduces constipation. Approximately 20 gram of it its juice should be taken, which is better with other mixtures.

16. Grape Juice

Vitamins A, B, C, potassium, iron and other minerals are found in it.

Through grape juice, one can get rid of cancer, gout, skin disease, ulcer, jaundice, plethora, acidity, blood pressure and stomach related problems.

It improves eye sight, purifies blood and increase vitality. It removes poisonous toxins from the body.

Consumption of grape juice is beneficial in asthma. It is also useful in treating migraine. Grape juice increases blood cells. During teething and constipation of children, giving grape juice is helpful. Its juice acts as a tonic for the kidney and liver. It has phytonutrient called Ellagic Acid, which stops swelling, cancer and high BP.

17. Lemon Juice

Lemon has most of the necessary vitamins, and minerals. It is beneficial for liver and stomach problems. It is also very helpful in treatment of brain-related problems and mental disorder. It has vitamin C in abundance and cleans the blood and stomach. It helps in reducing body fat, if taken with honey, in lukewarm water. It is beneficial in treating skin diseases specially itching and cold and cough. Lemon juice is also beneficial in dyptheria, typhoid and other fevers. Taking lemon juice with onion juice and water in the morning and evening, helps in preventing gas and indigestion. It can be used in all seasons.

Lemon juice improves appetite. It breaks down kidney stones. It is useful in asthma and jaundice.

18. Margosa Leaves Juice

Every day, on an empty stomach, taking ½-2 teaspoon of margosa leaves juice, purifies the blood, improves the skin complexion and strengthens the liver. This prescription is also effective in treating cough, fever and patients of diabetes.

19. Mint Juice

It has abundance of vitamin A along with vitamins B, C, D and E. Apart from this there is also calcium, phosphorus and iron mineral elements. Mint juice performs the function of stimulating the act of digestion. Consumption of mint juice mixed with lemon juice relieves the pain of gas immediately. Mint is very useful for removing the worms in the stomach. It is beneficial in treating cold, cough, asthma and low digestion. At one time, 30 grams of juice is sufficient, which can be taken with other mixtures.

20. Orange Juice

Orange is predigested food just like honey. It is a good source of providing energy to tired people.

By taking orange juice early in the morning, constipation and digestion related problems are removed. Orange juice contains sugar, because of which it gives activeness to weak people. To increase life force, orange juice should be taken twice in a day.

If a pregnant woman has an orange daily, then the child born will be healthy. Children who are not brought up on mother's milk should definitely be given orange juice. This food protects them from scurvy and rickets. Orange juice acts as medicine in diseases like pyorrhoea, high BP, obesity, fever, influenza, anaemia, asthma, cold, diabetes, rheumatisms and insomnia.

It has vitamins A, B and C in abundance. It keeps the liver free from disease and makes it strong. It benefits people suffering from skin diseases and mental diseases.

It works like a tonic for small children. During teething of a child, orange juice serves the purpose of medicine.

Orange juice provides mental energy too. Its phytonutrients are believed to protect humans from cancer.

21. Raw Papaya Juice

This is an excellent source of relief from heat. It is beneficial for those who have bad digestion problems. Raw papaya juice is very good for removing skin diseases. Menstruation related problems are removed through consumption of raw papaya juice. This juice lessens the swelling, cleans the intestines and melts and removes tumors present.

22. Pear Juice

Pear juice is completely digestible. Being sweet, it is also a good beverage. If constipation patients consume pear juice for two-three days, then constipation, indigestion, etc., are removed. Drinking pear juice leads to mucus in faeces some times, but one should not get worried by this. This mucus develops because of the stomach getting cleaned. It stops within 2-3 days.

Pear juice is beneficial in diabetes, ulcer, eczema, gout, piles and colitis. It gives strength to the heart, brain, stomach and liver. Its juice is helpful in removing stones and increases vitality. It has a phytonutrient named Quercetin which reduces swelling and allergy.

23. Pineapple Juice

Pineapple juice is especially beneficial in dyptheria and throat problems. It is a store house of iodine, phosphoric acid, iron, magnesium, sodium, potassium and vitamins A, B and C. Pineapple juice has the quality of being able to remove mucus from the intestines. It is especially beneficial in lung diseases, indigestion, constipation, jaundice and chronic disease of the stomach.

It is helpful in killing germs of the stomach and has the capacity of helping digest protein. It helps in removing body swelling. It is beneficial in fever, skin problem and diabetes. It cures cough, helps in liver problem and is beneficial in urinary disease. It is very effective in removing stones of the kidney. It removes pimples and blood disorders. It also helps in asthma, rheumatism, gout, etc., when taken, as one bowl juice mixed with one spoon honey. Its juice can be taken after mixing with water. It has a phytonutrient called Bromelanin which prevents blood clot formation. It also has a phytonutrient named Zingiberone which is very beneficial in rheumatoid arthritis. It also has antioxidants.

24. Pomegranate Juice

Pomegranate juice is a good treatment for the worms of the stomach. It has high quality sodium. It also has sufficient amounts of iron, Vitamin C and tanic acid. Pomegranate juice acts quickly in health improvement. Its juice is very beneficial in diarrhoea, sprue and anaemia. It improves the working capacity of liver and intestines. It effects well immediately in jaundice, high BP, rheumatism, piles and bleeding of gums. Nettlerash is suppressed by mixing and taking pomegranate juice mixed with honey.

25. Potato Juice

Potato juice is quite cheap and we also get a good quantity of nutrition from it. It contains Vitamin A, B, C, minerals, chlorine, phosphorous, sulphur, potassium and other nutrients. It gives a lot of relief from stomach diseases like ulcer. Its protein is of good and high quality. It is also very effective for gout, kidney stones, skin diseases, etc. It gives relief from heart burn and back ache. It removes constipation. Its Solanin, a phytonutrient, decreases swelling and removes rheumatoid arthritis and also decreases the problems of the nervous system.

26. Radish Juice

It is beneficial in diabetes and heart problem. It digests food, removes acidity, benefits in urinary diseases and destroys cough.

This juice is very pungent, hence should be taken after mixing with other juices. This juice, when taken along with carrot juice removes mucus.

27. Spinach Juice

Spinach is most popular among leafy vegetables. It is grown in all places and available throughout the year. It has abundance of Vitamins B and E. It also has iron, potassium, sodium and amino acid.

If one glass of spinach juice is given to a malnutritioned child daily, than it is very beneficial. Spinach has a lot of folic acid, therefore pregnant women must take this for development of the foetus.

If spinach juice is given along with raw coconut then because of having nitrate and potassium, it works as a diuretic. Regular consumption of spinach juice removes constipation. It strengthens the teeth and gums. Pyorrhoea patients must eat spinach. It increases eyesight.

Spinach juice is very good for cleansing of intestines.

For breast feeding women, consumption of spinach juice is very helpful.

It should definitely be given in case of anaemia and jaundice.

Its regular consumption removes pimples. Is very good for stomach ulcer. Its phytonutrients prevents ageing, cancer, cataract and sight weakness.

28. Sweet Lemon Juice

Sweet lemon is an energy-giving, tasty fruit. It is helpful in removing anaemia and improves digestion. Toxins which get accumulated in the digestive tract gets cleaned easily by this juice.

Its juice is beneficial for patients with skin problems. It is a good source of Vitamin C, calcium and phosphorous. It is very effective in liver diseases and mental imbalance.

29. Tomato Juice

Tomato has potassium and iron and hence it is helpful in curing skin diseases and keeps the skin beautiful and healthy.

It is very effective in treating jaundice, indigestion, diseased liver, constipation and chronic sinus. It has vitamins A, B and C in abundance. It has citric acid, phosphoric acid and melic acid and is therefore good for physical and mental health. It is very important for anaemia. Along with increasing blood, it also purifies the blood.

It kills the germs of the stomach and increases appetite. It's regular consumption makes the face glow and pre-ejaculation, leucorrhoea, sagging of breast, etc., do not occur. Tomato juice is beneficial for children's growth. In this, antioxidants are found which improve health. It has a phytonutrient called Lycopene which is helpful in cancer and heart diseases.

30. Turnip Juice

Turnip juice is beneficial for health. Turnip has a good amount of calcium and vitamin C. As it has sufficient calcium, so it is good for teeth and bones. Turnip juice, being slightly salty, should be taken mixed with lemon juice. Its regular consumption helps in cough also. It has phytonutrients named Indoles and Sulphoraphane which prevents cancer.

31. Watermelon Juice

Along with being tasty, it is also improves health. It has a lot of vitamins A, B and C. It also has calcium, phosphorus, potassium, iron and magnesium minerals in sufficient quantity. It is the best beverage to prevent effect of heat and to bring about activeness. It is helpful in reducing the body's acidity. It removes urinary diseases. It is also very beneficial in joint pain, blood pressure and treating stones of kidney. Watermelon juice is a good tonic. It also reduces mental stress. It has a phytonutrient named Lycopene which prevents cancer and heart diseases.

32. Wheat Grass Juice

It has been scientifically researched and proved that wheat grass juice improves life force, which leads to a disease free future. Due to its endless qualities, it cannot be compared to any other thing, thus it has also been named as an ambrosial nectar. Due to its special qualities it has been given high place in research.

This juice has the excellent capacity of dissolving and removing settled poisonous waste from the intestines and blood. Due to its power of removing toxins from the body, it has been said to be very efficacious medicine for all human diseases.

From wheat grass juice, carbohydrate, protein, all vitamins, high quality alkaline nutrients, enzymes and chlorophyll are found in a natural way. This chlorophyll strengthens the heart, makes blood circulation easy and specially benefits intestines, lungs and uterus.

If a pregnant woman takes wheat grass juice regularly during pregnancy then it will greatly benefit her child. If a sterile woman keeps taking this juice, then it improves her chances of pregnancy. If 5 drops of it are given to a child regularly then he remains healthy and sound.

By taking wheat grass juice and ideal natural food, all diseases are removed.

Wheat grass juice treatment is definitely beneficial in incurable diseases, gas, acidity, diabetes, anaemia, worms, Parkinson's, skin disease, kidney stone, menstrual irregularity, heart problem and cancer.

Its application on gums give special benefit and its consumption removes teeth and gum diseases. It is good for constipation. It regulates the weight of a person. Its juice helps in all diseases and acts like a tonic.

33. White Pumpkin Juice

White pumpkin is completely alkaline. It has iron, calcium, sulphur, phosphorous minerals and vitamins A, B and C. It cures nettlerash. It removes acid from the body and removes swelling and burning sensations. It is a sure way to cure constipation.

Its consumption cures piles, bleeding piles, and ulcer. Its juice is also beneficial in tuberculosis. It removes urinary diseases and also removes heat of the liver. Jaundice is also removed.

It cures the burning sensation in stomach and lungs and also removes swelling of the food pipe. It is beneficial in epilepsy and all the diseases related to nervous system. It must surely be used for purpose of killing worms of the intestine. It is very important in blood pressure disease. It is very beneficial in angina. It must be used by asthmatic patients, especially who use inhalers.

It is also very good for leucorrhoea. It removes the stones of kidney, urinary bladder and gall bladder. It is also very effective in treating impotency, sterility and leucorrhoea. It has a phytonutrient named Lycopene which stops the harmful effect of heart disease, cancer of prostate, early ageing and diabetes.

Various Combination of Juices

Juice of fruits and vegetables are undoubtedly very tasty, healthy and full of medicinal value in their individual form but for new tastes and more effective medicinal values, different combinations can be made.

1. Carrot 3 portion, tomato 2 portion, beetroot 1 portion. Taking this juice everyday removes wrinkles of face, pigmentation and pimples and worms from stomach is removed. Face starts glowing. It is also good in acidity.
2. Carrot 250 gram, beetroot 75 gram, amla 50 gram, raw turmeric 25 gram and ginger 5 gram. Taking this juice everyday stops early ageing.

3. Juice of carrot 5 portion, beetroot 1 portion and cabbage 1 portion, helps in acidity and ulcer.
4. Mixture of 1 glass tomato juice, 8-10 crushed mint leaves and juice of half lemon, gives relief from constipation, worms of stomach and pimples. Skin becomes fair.
5. Mix juice of 2 amla, one teaspoon honey in one glass of water. It is tasty and nutritious. It is beneficial in diabetes, constipation, blood impurities and urinary related diseases.
6. Taking mixture of carrot 3 portion and spinach 1 portion, increases physical-mental strength and eyesight. It also helps in piles.
7. Drink the mixture of raw turmeric 50 gram, ginger 50 gram, one teaspoon honey in one glass of water. This keeps ageing away and strengthen the liver. It purifies blood. Reduces the swelling of body parts and is also beneficial in cold and cough.
8. Make the juice of 300 gram carrot, 100 gram tomato, 50 gram beetroot, a little coriander juice and add juice of half a lemon to it. This is good for anaemia, skin diseases, obesity and diabetes. It is especially beneficial for pregnant women. It is also extremely good for eyes.
9. Juice of 300 gram bottle gourd, 300 gram cucumber, 10 gram ginger, 15 basil leaves, and 15 gram coriander leaves is especially useful for heart disease and high BP.
10. Make the juice of cabbage, carrot, beetroot, spinach, tomato and amla in equal proportion. This is especially good for winter diseases.
11. Make the juice of white pumpkin, bottle gourd and tomato in equal proportion. This is especially good for summer diseases.
12. Take the juice of 300 gram carrot, 3 gram cabbage, 200 gram bottle gourd and 200 gram white pumpkin. This is especially useful for stomach diseases and gout.
13. Make the juice of 60% green leaves (spinach, fenugreek, coriander, mint, etc.), 25% bottle gourd or white

pumpkin, cucumber, cabbage, 15% tomato and little ginger. Mix lemon juice to it and consume. This is generally beneficial in all diseases, specially diabetes, cancer and constipation. It works as a tonic for liver and eyes.

Extremely tasty other combinations

1. One bowl apple juice + 1 bowl sweet lime juice.
2. One bowl apple juice + ½ bowl cherry juice + 2 teaspoon ginger juice.
3. One bowl pineapple juice + one bowl grapes juice + one spoon honey.
4. One part pineapple juice + one part grape juice + one part sweet lime juice + one part apple juice.

Juice Fasting

Fasting is a good source of maintaining health and rebuilding lost health. Therefore fasting is necessary both for a sick as well as normal person.

In juice fasting, only the juice of fruits and vegetable is taken. Juice fasting is the best way of fasting.

Removing inner toxins of the body is the primary function of fasting. This act is speeded up by juices.

Fruits

Fruit is a wonderful gift of nature. Religion, holy books, Vedas, Upanishads and Puran, all have described and worshipped the fruit diet in one way or another. The Holy Koran has also described various fruits like grape, date, fig and pomegranate. Similarly The Holy Bible too has descriptions of fruits. In ancient time, man made the maximum use of fruits. Being in nature's courtyard, man used to spend a healthy, happy and long life. However, when man started indulging in unnatural and pompous life styles, fruits diet remained only for namesake and its place was taken by disease-causing cooked food, meat, fish and fried materials. As a result, man started going from a healthy to unhealthy life.

Fruit works both as food and as medicine.

From treatment point of view, fruits hold an important place. Taking medicines later on gives birth to one or more diseases, whereas getting rid of disease through fruits guarantees safety from disease in the future.

Even the most incurable diseases are cured by it. On the Central Nervous System being unhealthy, it is impossible for a person to remain healthy. But fruits have a protective and strengthening effect on the nervous system and the person remains healthy. One who takes fruits regularly has sharp intelligence and does not get easily tired working and as a result he remains free from mental tension and is not effected by weakness and impotency. One attains completeness in spiritual practice. Fruits are essential for intelligent people, people of old age and spiritual practitioners. Use of regional and seasonal fruits is preferable as they are grown naturally according to the climate and requirement of the body.

Fruits

1. Apple

Apple has A, B, C and E vitamins and iron, phosphorus, potassium, etc. It strengthens the brain and sharpens intelligence and removes nervous weakness. It cleans the stomach. Apple has an important role in removing mental irritability, decreased vitality and laziness. It is helpful in anaemia. It is beneficial in both constipation and diarrhoea. It is very good for heart patients. It is also a diurectic to remove toxins. Its antioxidants reduce cholesterol. It is like a nectar for people living in hilly areas. It has a phytonutrient named Phenolic Compounds which stops heart problems.

2. Banana

Vitamins A, B, D, E and minerals, calcium, iron, potassium, phosphorus, etc., are found in abundance in ripe bananas. It is not only an easily digestible food but is also like medicine for removing many diseases. It increases weight of children and cures the digestive power of weak people. It controls high BP. It removes acidity and ulcer of the stomach. Its antioxidants remove the deposited uric acid in joint pain. It is a good medicine for heart problem. It helps a lot in leucorrhoea.

The inner portion of a banana peel should definitely be eaten as it has many natural salts.

Identification of ripe banana—1) Should be spotty. 2) Banana should break on being lifted from the bunch and not by pulling it with force, 3) should be easily peeled, 4) should not be oily in eating, instead should be very sweet and dissoluble in mouth.

Note – Half ripe bananas should be kept covered with cloth or paper in a basket and consumed on becoming spotty.

3. Black Berry

Black berry has many nutritious elements. It is very good in Kapha and Pitta problems. Eating black berries makes the teeth and gums healthy. Diabetes patient should regularly eat black berries. It is beneficial in stomach diseases. Black berries' juice give relief in stone problems. It removes heart problem and leprosy. It strengthens the stomach, pancreas and spleen. Black berries purifies blood and prevents urinary diseases. Its antioxidants have good capacity of removing toxins from the human body. It is very useful in treating an enlarged liver. It works like a tonic on the heart and nerves. It gives relief in bleeding piles condition.

The Anthocyanins present in it stops ageing. It also has Ellagic acid which reduces cholesterol and helps in preventing cancer.

Only ripe and fresh black berries should be eaten. It should not be combined with milk or curd. If one has eaten too many mangoes then eating black berries act as a digestive agent. Black berries should not be eaten too many at a time.

4. Cherry

It is nutritious, a blood enhancer and constipation remover. It has abundant vitamins A and C. It is good for diabetes and heart patient. It has same phytonutrients as in blue berries.

5. Custard Apple

It has iron, carbohydrate, calcium, phosphorus, vitamin A, etc. It is a blood enhancer, good for the heart, strength enhancer and Pitta dosha destroyer. Its pulp is especially helpful in nervous diseases. Cleans stomach and is beneficial in gout.

6. Grape

It has vitamins A, B, C, etc., calcium, phosphorus, iron, potassium and carbohydrate in abundance.

It removes constipation, cures kidney problems, helps in gout, jaundice, anaemia, enlarged liver, spleen disease and also increases weight.

Sweet grapes prevent cancer, anaemia, stones of kidney and tuberculosis. It is nutritious and a strength enhancer. It increases eye sight and appetite and helps produce new

Fruits

blood cells. It is a very good food source during pregnancy. It should be taken by mothers who have less milk production. It removes colitis and old constipation. It is beneficial in heart problem. It has a phytonutrient named Bio Flavonoids which quickly removes toxins from the body.

7. Falsa

Falsa removes dirty waste from the body. It removes dryness and heat of the brain. It strengthens heart, stomach and liver. It is also helpful in burning sensation while passing urine and leucorrhoea. Juice of falsa is beneficial in Pitta dosha and heart disease.

8. Guava

It has abundant vitamins A, C, etc., and minerals, calcium, iron, phosphorus, etc. To have a beautiful child it is very useful before pregnancy, during pregnancy and after delivery while feeding the child. It prevents stone of gall bladder, strengthens the teeth and removes swelling of the gums. It kills germs of the stomach and increases appetite. It removes constipation and completely cleans the intestines. Its consumption removes many toxins from the stomach. It acts like a tonic for the liver and removes blood impurities. It is helpful in strengthening the nerves. Guava should neither be too ripe nor too raw.

9. Jujube/Zizyphus

It is useful in diarrhoea, gout and gas problem. I's regular consumption avoids constipation and stone of urinary bladder. It improves vitality, appetite and eyesight. It destroys tuberculosis.

10. Loquat

It has calcium, phosphorus, iron, etc., and vitamin A. It is beneficial in treating bleeding piles, low memory power and stiffness of the liver.

11. Mango

It is believed to be the best fruit of the world. The mango which falls from the branch after being ripe is said to be the best. Ripe mango has useful contents like protein, fat, carbohydrate, potassium, calcium, iron, phosphorus, etc., and vitamins A, B, and C. It is gas destroyer, improves muscles and vitality and provides strength. It is blood purifier and blood enhancer. It increases digestive power. Removes weakness of the kidney; gives strength to heart and liver.

It increases weight of weak people. It removes semen weakness, impotency and night falls. It is also very useful is tuberculosis. The Beta Carotene present in it removes signs of ageing, prevents cancer, develops lungs and stops harmful effect of diabetes.

Note –
1. One should not eat raw and too ripe mango.
2. Before eating mangoes they should be put in water for 1-2 hours.
3. Eating too much mangoes lead to blood disorder, constipation and gas.

12. Mulberry

It has elements like calcium, iron, phosphorous, etc., and vitamins A, C, etc. It cures cough, helps blood production and destroys worms in the stomach and improves digestive power. It is useful in treating cold and throat diseases. It is very useful in Pitta dosha and blood disorder.

13. Melon

It has all useful elements important for life, carotene and vitamin A in abundance. Regular consumption of melon during its season keeps a person healthy. After child birth, if a mother consumes melon (during season) then the quantity of breast milk increases. Pulp of ripe melon provides strength to the heart. It helps in all skin diseases specially eczema. It pacifies pain of Pitta Dosha and Vata Dosha, removes urine problem, stomach infection and destroys gas.

14. Orange

Orange is the most widely used fruit from the health and taste point of view. Its juice has vitamin C, iron, potassium, calcium, phosphorous and sugar in sufficient amounts. It is very beneficial for children, old people and patients. It dissolves the toxins, increases amount of urine and thus removes waste from the body. It increases resistance power for infectious diseases. Consuming orange, normally and regularly during season, definitely prevents cold, gum disease, piles and unnatural bleeding and the person becomes strong and robust. Its juice is beneficial for the liver and heart. If taken with honey in heart problems, it becomes even more beneficial. If 1-2 spoon amla juice is added to it, then its benefits increase.

Eating oranges reduces mental stress and irritability. If a pregnant woman feels nauseated, then having an orange gives immediate relief. Weak children should regularly take oranges.

The Hesperitin present in it stops the increasing number of cancer cells and prevents mouth cancer. Normally people hesitate to take oranges during colds or heart diseases but there is no logic to it. Orange is beneficial in all ways. It has abundant vitamin C which is a protective vitamin and cold and cough remains away through this.

15. Papaya

This has a very high quality of the digestive element, papain. Various vitamin and minerals are found in it. Its regular consumption eliminates chances of stone. It keeps the stomach clean. It strengthens the liver. It increases breast milk in lactating women. It is beneficial in gas problem, high BP, constipation, piles and gout. It increases appetite. Ripe papaya is taken as a fruit and raw papaya is used in juice form.

The Beta Carotene present in it acts as an anti ageing agent, prevents from cancer, develops lungs and stops the harmful effect of diabetes.

16. Peach

This has vitamins A, B, C, etc., and minerals calcium, phosphorous, iron, and potassium in abundance. It removes constipation and stone of urinary bladder. It stops the production of worms in the stomach.

17. Pear

Other fruits of this species are Naakh and Baboogosha. It gives strength to heart, brain, stomach and liver. It destroys Vatta, Pitta and Kapha. It has almost all the natural elements in some or more quantity. It is useful in stone of kidney and gall bladder. Due to its high quality of diuretic, it helps in gout and pain in urination. It removes constipation and is semen enhancer.

The Quercetins present in it reduces swelling along with allergy. It stops further increase of head and neck tumour and protects the lungs from harmful effects of pollution.

18. Pineapple

Pineapple is a health giving, pleasant fruit. It has many qualities. Removes uneasiness, quenches thirst, keeps the body healthy and provides freshness. It gives strength to the heart and brain. Eating pineapple on an empty stomach improves digestion. Makes urination proper and thus helps prevent stones. It is helpful in swelling of throat and tonsillitis. It is also beneficial in thyroid problem.

The Bromelanin present in it prevents clotting of blood. The Chlorogenic Acid present in it acts as an antioxidant.

19. Plum/Prune

Plum is full of nutritious elements. It is a good source of iron and potassium. High antioxidants present in it, reduces the effect of heart disease, lung problem, cancer, cataract and old age. It is especially helpful in constipation. It is very good for pregnant and breast feeding women. It prevents weakness of bones in women after menopause. It is also a diuretic. Similar to mango, this too has a phytonutrient named Beta Carotene.

20. Pomegranate

This has abundant protein, vitamin and natural salts, required and necessary for life. Its important antioxidant prevents cancer and heart problem. It reduces cholesterol, increases appetite, gives quick relief in jaundice, and help in formation of blood.

21. Raspberry

Juicy and tasty, raspberry is a useful source of Vitamins A, C and minerals, potassium, iron, etc. It prevents tuberculosis, heart disease and cancer. The Luetin, Myricertin and Quercetins present in it prevent cancer, heart and lung diseases.

22. Sapota

It has abundant sugar, phosphorous, iron and potassium. It is anti-constipation. Regular consumption with honey improves sexual prowess and removes pre-ejaculation.

23. Strawberry

It contains a high quality of zinc, which is necessary for semen. It has high quality folic acid which is necessary for pregnant women. It is also very useful in treating eczema and asthma. The Anthocyanins present in it acts as an anti ageing agent. It also has Ellagic Acid which reduces cholesterol and stops cancer.

24. Sweet Lemon

Its nutritive and medicinal values are same as that of an orange. Only the taste and smell are different. Other fruits of this species like Malta and Kinnu also have the same qualities. It is a blood purifier and digestive. It is a health improver and

increases activeness. It is beneficial in skin diseases.
Secret of Health Uncooked Food

25. *Watermelon*

This is very useful for us and is cheap and easily available. It has more water than any other fruit. This water has abundant potassium which dissolves toxins present in the body and removes it through urine/sweat. It is the best diuretic hence helps specially in urination disturbance, lack of urine, stone of kidney and urinary bladder, increase uric acid and calcium in urine. It also helps in reducing obesity.

Excess sweating in summers leads to loss of natural salt and makes one feel thirsty, but eating watermelon not only quenches thirst but also provides natural salt and protects us from harmful effect of heat (sun rays). The Lycopene present in it prevents heart disease and prostate cancer.

Vegetables

Vegetables are medicines as well as excellent tonics. These have the valuable quality of increasing body immunity.

It is best to consume vegetables in raw form. These have necessary vitamin and minerals. These have very high quality of antioxidants which removes toxins from the body very quickly. They are digestive and anti-constipation.

1. Beetroot

Beetroot is usually eaten as a salad. Its consumption brings glow to the face. It cleans the small intestine and removes constipation. It purifies blood. It regulates the functioning of blood production. Blood pressure remains controlled. If someone's hands and legs have cracks in winter, then taking beetroot prevents them. Taking beetroot helps in women's diseases, irregularity of menstrual cycle and leucorrhoea. Removes pigmentation of skin and blackness of nails and they become healthy. Eating raw beetroot with honey is the cheapest source of high quality nutrition.

The Betanin present in it prevents cancer and heart diseases.

2. Cabbage

As long as cabbage is available, it should definitely be eaten raw in form of salad. It has a high quality of calcium. It has abundant vitamin U which is the nutritive substance for protecting the inner layer of the stomach. It removes the ulcer of stomach, swelling of the liver, jaundice, bleeding of gums, piles, heart disease and excessive acidity in urine. It has many types of phytonutrients which also stops cancer.

3. Carrot

Carrot has nutritive elements for the body. It has vitamins B, C, D, E and A in abundance. It also has potassium, calcium, phosphorus, sulphur and sodium in abundance. Carrot is famous for its nutritive qualities. It is also very beneficial for the eyes. It is useful for skin disease, tuberculosis, nervous weakness, cancer, toxaemia and constipation.

Chewing carrot, after eating food, kills the harmful germs of the mouth and makes the teeth strong and clean. It stops gum bleeding.

It removes chronic and severe constipation and removes smell of bad breath. Its regular consumption stops the possibility of peptic ulcer, cancer and other disease of the digestive system. It is very useful in treating urinary tract stones. It improves vitality. Mixing it with honey further enhances, its qualities.

It has phytonutrients called Beta Carotene which is anti-ageing, prevents from cancer, develops the lungs and stops the harmful effects of diabetes.

4. Cucumber

It is alkaline and is also a blood purifier. It is also beneficial in stone diseases. It cures constipation and is helpful for obesity, gout, diabetes and kidney problems. It eliminates cough and is most effective in reducing weight. It is useful in urinary disturbance and fever. Cucumber must be eaten raw and fresh.

5. Garlic

Garlic is of two varieties- one with many cloves and one with one clove. The one with single clove has more importance. It has volatile oil (smell) and is also a useful enzyme. Due to its pungent smell it has the quality of destroying germs. In winters, garlic produces heat in the body. It increases sexual power and reduces high BP. It is beneficial in tuberculosis. It is useful in asthma, cough and paralysis. It reduces cholesterol.

On an empty stomach, 2-3 cloves should be eaten by chewing properly and then water should be taken afterwards. It can be taken by grinding it and mixing with honey and water. It can be used in various chutneys. The Allium Compounds present in it prevents from cancer and reduce high BP and cholesterol.

6. Onion

Onion has the same qualities as that of garlic. It is digestive, increases appetite and removes constipation. It removes problems arising out of change in climate. It helps in treating stomach problem, acidity and sour burp. It increases sexual power in men. It protects from sunstroke. It cures insomnia. To remove the smell of onion —
1. After eating onion, eat one fresh fruit such as apple, peach, pear, etc.
2. Before eating onion, dip them in salty water.
3. Eat one small piece of lemon.
4. Gargle with mixture of lemon juice and rose water.
5. Chew mint leaves.

7. Peas

Eating raw peas in the form of salad, removes many diseases from our body. Fresh peas contain calcium, phosphorus, sulphur and iron in abundant quantity. This purifies blood, improves muscles, and gives new energy to heart and lungs. Digestive power is improved and constipation is removed.

8. Radish

Radish has several vitamins and minerals amongst which iron, sodium and potassium are in abundance. Radish is very useful in dissolving stone. It also removes urine problems. The pungent smell of radish destroys the worms of stomach and work as a strong antibiotic. Radish cleans the stomach, removes constipation and takes out toxins from the body. Radish strengthens the bone and teeth. It is also very useful in piles, jaundice and leucoderma.

Radish leaves should be eaten along with it. One should not combine milk or curd with radish.

9. Tomato

Tomato is nutritive as well as a medicine for many diseases. It has vitamin and minerals in abundance. It increases red blood cell. It increases digestive power and appetite and is an energy enhancer. Eating 2-3 ripe tomatoes regularly quickens the growth of children. Regular consumption of tomatoes keeps the stomach clean. Eating tomato with ground black pepper in the morning, on an empty stomach helps to remove worms of the stomach. If one gets blisters in the mouth too often then he should eat more tomatoes. Tomatoes act like a medicine for blisters. The Lycopene present in it reduces cholesterol and prevents many type of cancer.

Note – Tomato should neither be too raw nor too ripe.

10. Turnip

It has vitamins A, B, C and iron, sulphur, potassium and calcium. It destroys cough and reduces uric acid in the urine. The Indoles and Sulphoraphane, prevents from various cancer.

11. Vegetable Marrow

It can grow a few inches long or up to 3 feet. During summers it reduces intensity of blood and Pitta dosha. It keeps the body cool. Removes the burning sensation of urine. It is beneficial in stone of kidney, diabetes, gout and urine disease. It is digestive hence helps in indigestion.

Leafy Vegetables

Green leafy vegetables are the excellent gift of nature which not only give us taste but also keeps our body healthy and develop the capacity to fight with diseases. They have all the minerals, calcium, sodium, iron and chlorine in abundance. They also have extra roughage, some carbohydrates and proteins. For example carrot leaves have four times more iron and calcium then carrot, beetroot leaves has 15 times more iron and calcium than beetroot, radish leaves has 3 times more iron and 15 times more calcium as compared to radish. These are store house of vitamin and chlorophyll. On occurrence of a disease, instead of eating artificial capsules of vitamin, calcium or iron, the leafy vegetables work as the best medicine. Their usage make the disease disappear in the same manner as darkness disappears by sunrise. Leafy vegetables should be thoroughly washed in running water and should be eaten raw. These are available throughout the year and both the rich and poor can get it easily. They can also be produced in kitchen gardens.

1. Bengal Gram Leaves

Bengal gram leaves has iron, calcium and phosphorus in abundance. In season, eating bengal gram leaves daily, prevent tooth decay. It also helps in pyorrhoea. It is useful for liver, lungs, spleen, swelling of bones and eye diseases.

2. Broccoli

This is a green vegetable similar to cauliflower. The antioxidant Glucosinoletes is very effective in stopping cancer. It increases resistance power. It is eaten raw in form of salad. It has many phytonutrients such as Sulphoraphane, Indoles, Beta Carotene, Luetin and Quercetins, which prevents ageing, cancer, harmful effect of cataract and diabetes and damage of muscles. They reduce swelling along with allergy.

3. Celery

It improves digestion, cures cough, benefits the heart, improves vitality, and is an energiser. It removes eye disease. The 3-n-butyl Parthalid present in it reduces high BP, and Luetin prevents cataract.

4. Coriander Leaves

These have a high quality fragrance. It removes bad smell. Its consumption removes bad smell of onion too. It removes Pitta Dosha. Green coriander can be eaten with salad. It should always be used fresh and in small quantity.

5. Drum Stick Leaves

It is the treasure throve of vitamin A. It is the storehouse of amino acid, potassium, calcium, and iron. It enhances semen, is beneficial for eyes and heart and destroys cough and worms.

6. Fenugreek Leaves

Fenugreek leaves has minerals like iron, calcium, etc., in good quantity and vitamin C and carotene as well.

7. Ipomoea

It is very useful for patients of constipation. It has iron and iodine in abundance. It improves intelligence. It destroys cough and swelling. Its consumption makes the hair strong and black. It is useful in goitre and anaemia.

8. Lettuce

It has various vitamins and minerals. It prevents cancer and increases immunity. It is digestive and destroys constipation.

The Quercetins present in it stops cancer, reduces swelling along with allergy. It prevents the growth of head and neck tumour. It protects the lungs from the harmful effect of pollution.

9. Mint

Mint is a digestive, appetiser, kills worms and bad smell, heart strengthener, diuretic, pain remover, helper in skin diseases and wounds healer.

Consuming fresh mint leaves daily works as an effective germ destroyer and teeth protector. It prevents tooth decay, pyorrhoea and early falling off of teeth. Eating this with figs, removes the accumulated cough in the chest and stops hiccups. Chewing 8-10 mint leaves removes gas. It should be eaten raw to keep its vitamins intact.

10. Radish Leaves

Radish leaves has iron and calcium in abundance. It also has vitamins in sufficient quantity. While eating radish, its leaves should also be eaten. Leaves improve digestion of radish and remove gas problem.

11. Spinach

Spinach has the required amino acid, calcium, iron, vitamins A, C and folic acid. During summers, spinach can be eaten by mixing in salad. Regular consumption of iron during pregnancy removes iron deficiency, uterus bleeding, miscarriage and loose motions. It improves physical development, health and eyesight, thus feeding spinach to children is very useful. It is also helpful in increasing quality of milk of breast feeding mothers.

On having constipation, spinach leaves should be eaten in bulk. Eating raw spinach with honey helps in cough and respiratory disease.

For those children who get low nutrition, eating fresh spinach regularly is a god's gift. It increases the resistance power of the body.

The Zeathanxin present in it prevents cancer of large intestine.

12. White Goose Poot (Bathua)

It has iron, phosphorous, calcium in abundance. It increases appetite. It improves quality of semen and strength. It is very useful for liver, spleen, eye disease, piles, obesity, worm disease, indigestion, stomach problems and normal weakness. It prevents all the diseases of urination. It can be eaten by mixing in salad. It removes pre-ejaculation and impotency. It is especially beneficial in heart disease.

Sprouted Food

Sprouted food is very important for physical, mental and spiritual balance. Sprouts do not merely remain grain but its starch gets converted to glucose and its protein into amino acid thus becoming easily digestive, healthy and energy enhancing that is why it is also called predigested food.

Sprouted food is a good source of chlorophyll, vitamin (A, B, C, D and K, etc.), calcium, phosphorous, potassium, magnesium, iron, etc. It has necessary enzymes for health, antioxidants and phyto chemicals.

Sprouted food increases appetite, removes poisonous elements from the body and improves urination.

Sprouted food is complete food and can make a person young again and keeps a person healthy beautiful and disease free.

Sprout is a good source of giving instant energy to the body. It is quickly and easily absorbed by the body.

Sprout removes malnutrition.

Sprout food destroys gas and constipation.

Sprout is a food to cure diseases. Sprout can take place of expensive fruits and vegetables. It is cheap and easy to prepare. Thus it can be according to everybody's budget.

It does not have any adulteration.

Sprout food is also helpful in getting rid of addictions.

What to Sprout

Wheat, moong, moth, soyabean, groundnut, maize, sesame, gram, alfalfa, sunflower seeds and other grains, pulses, seeds, etc.

Method of making sprout

Dry food grain, pulse or seed, etc., whatever has to sprouted should be washed and soaked in a bowl of water.

Use luke warm water in winters. After 12 hours take out from water and keep in cloth so that they get air and moisture. Keep sprinkling water many times on it during summers to keep them damp. Within 12-30 hours (according to different foods) germination will start.

When the sprout is ready, wash and use. In this process some seeds which are not sprouted should be taken out and removed.

How to Eat Sprout

1. It is best to eat sprouted food raw, uncooked and without salt.
2. Along with single grains (wheat, maize, jowar, bajra, etc.) sweet food (dates, raisin, black raisin, honey etc.) and fruits can be taken.
3. Grains which can be split (gram, moong, moth, peas, groundnut, soya bean, etc.) can be eaten with tomato, carrot, cucumber, vegetable marrow, capsicum, green leaves (spinach, mint, coriander, white goose poot, etc.) and other salads and lemon juice. This mixture is very tasty and healthy.
4. For infants, children and old people, grind the sprout or the mixture to paste and then slowly make them lick it.
5. Eat the sprout raw only, because on cooking its nutritive value and goodness decreases.

Note – Wheat and sunflower sprout's size is as big as the seed, pulses sprout is double the seed and alfalfa sprout is best at 1-3 cm.

Alfalfa

Nature has given many rare substances to man and alfalfa is one of them. It is also known as Rizka or Lursen. The usage of this extraordinary grain, which is full of many life giving elements for the nutrition of human body is not fully known.

Sprouted alfalfa is very healthy. It has vitamins A, B, C, D, and E in sufficient amount. It is a store house of iron, calcium and phosphorus. It is especially beneficial for bones, formation of teeth and for the brain.

It also has many important antioxidants and phytonutrients.

Method of sprouting alfalfa

Wash the seed of alfalfa in plain water properly and soak in double water. After 4-6 hours, remove water and spread it on a linen cloth inside a basket with holes. Keep sprinkling water for dampness. After 3 days it starts germinating and after 6 days when the sprout is 1½-2" long then it is tasty to eat. If the sprouts become too long then it will not be tasty. Sprouted alfalfa increases 4-6 times in size. Its regular usage is very beneficial.

Dry Fruits

These have all the useful elements like carbohydrate, fat, protein, mineral salt, vitamin and roughage.

Eat walnut, cashewnut, pistachio nut, almond after soaking for 8 hours and throw out the water. Eat apricot and fig also after soaking and drink its water.

Almond

Regular consumption of almonds improves brain, nerves, bones, heart and function of liver. Almond has a very important natural element- copper. Almond is healthy and an energy giving food. Soaked almonds should be chewed properly for a long time while eating. Infants should be given paste of almond.

Cashewnut

It is a very tasty and useful food. It has high quality of protein. Dry cashewnut can increase cholesterol in the blood. Hence, it should be only eaten after being soaked. It strengthens the body and removes mental weakness.

Pistachio Nut

It is semen enhancer, blood purifier, energetic and cough destroyer. It removes three defects (Vata, Pitta, Kapha) of the body. It increases memory power and improves sexual power. Dry pistachio should be eaten after being soaked. In roasted pistachio most of the nutritious elements are destroyed. It has vitamin E in abundance and also sufficient amount of calcium.

Walnut

Along with being tasty it also has many qualities. It has high quality protein and potassium, magnesium, copper, zinc, vitamin B-6 and vitamin E are also found. It has the essential fat omega-3. It improves semen and gives energy. It removes heart disease and blood disorder. Eating walnut with honey removes tuberculosis, impotency and sterility. It strengthens the brain. Its regular usage improves memory power. Walnut is also very useful for diabetics. On consuming walnut, breast feeding mothers produce good amount of milk.

Apricot

Dry apricot has 6 times more calorie power than fresh fruit. Similarly in dry apricot, the quantity of carbohydrate, calcium and phosphorus also increases. It has vitamins A, B and C. Iron, calcium, phosphorous and potassium are found in abundance. It helps in digesting food. Having iron in abundance, it is very useful for anaemic patients. It prevents stone formation in gall bladder. It should be consumed after being soaked, along with its water. It destroys constipation, helpful in fever and is very good for skin. It has Beta Carotene which is anti-ageing, prevents cancer, develops lungs and stops the harmful effects of diabetes.

Fig

Fig has high quality Amino Acid, Tyurosine, Lysine and digestive enzyme, Protases. Eating fig with honey is very useful in tuberculosis, bleeding cough, asthma, bleeding piles, fistula and jaundice. It is helpful in stones and disease related to urine.

For improvement in growth of children, fig should be given since childhood. If a pregnant woman eats fig regularly, then she has easy delivery and does not feel weak afterwards.

It is very useful in digestion problem, constipation, cough, liver problem and sinusitis. It should be eaten after being soaked and its water must also be taken.

Natural Sweets

Dates, dry dates, raisin, black raisin, etc., are natural sweets which are full of nutrition and various minerals. These should be eaten after washing and soaking along with its water.

1. Dates

It is a cheap and energy giving natural sweet which is full of useful natural minerals like iron, calcium, phosphorus and potassium.

Dates give strength to stomach and heart, produces blood, makes the body fat and improves vital force. It is beneficial in dry cough and asthma. It removes swelling. It is useful in tuberculosis. In diabetes also where sweets is prohibited, one can have dates.

2. Dry Dates

It has calcium in abundance. Therefore eating this makes the bones strong, cures tooth decay and improves energy. It improves breathing problem, nervous weakness and blood circulation. It helps menstrual cycle. It is also useful in backache and stone. It is beneficial for children who bed wet and removes weakness of urination in old age. It improves sexual power.

3. Raisin

Raisin is excessively alkaline and is hence useful in maintaining alkaline and acidic balance of the body. It helps in constipation, anaemia, kidney and heart problems. Regularly eating 25 gram raisin improves glow of the face.

The Phenolic Compound present in it is very strong antioxidant which acts as an anti ageing agent.

4. Black Raisin

It gives energy, destroys constipation, helps in cold and cough, improves appetite, increases blood and enhances semen. It is full of various minerals and is a nutritious food.
Secret of Health Uncooked Food

Honey

Honey is like nectar for human beings. When a man becomes totally weak, voiceless and unconscious then at that time, on consuming honey, new life starts flowing within him. Honey is a predigested food, thus it immediately provides strength that is why there is the tradition of having honey from birth until death. It gets digested in only 5 minutes.

Honey has a very sweet taste. After milk, honey is the only such substance which comes under the category of good and balanced meal because honey has all those elements which should be present in a balanced food.

Honey has approximately 75% sugar among which fructose, glucose, sucrose, maltose and lactose are mainly present. Honey has 14 to 18 percent water in it. In form of other materials, protein, fat, enzymes and volatile aromatic materials are also present in sufficient amount. Not only this, honey also has vitamin A, B-1, B-2, B-3, B-5, B-6, B-12 along with small quantity of vitamin-C and K. Apart from this honey has iron, phosphorous, calcium and iodine.

Honey has been said to be like nectar in the Vedas and Puranas. There is no fixed time for having honey. It can be taken before meal, after meal or along with meal. It is not only food but is also a medicine.

Consolidation/Coagulation of Honey

Normally honey found from all type of sources can consolidate but some consolidate quickly and some slowly or after some years. Consolidation of honey is its special quality which depends on the various seasons and its source or flower. Some people in our society have misconception that honey which consolidates is fake but this misconception is baseless. Consolidated honey taste is much better and is full of all its important qualities. In winters it is also found in the honey bee's hive in consolidated form. Therefore while taking honey one should not pay attention towards its consolidation.

On putting the consolidated honey bottle in hot water it immediately comes back to liquid form.

Uses of Honey – Use of honey starts along with the beginning of human life. Just when the child is born he is given honey because consuming honey increases haemoglobin level, improves blood circulation, strengthens heart and along with this it gets mixed in the blood system due to which required energy is received immediately.

1. When a child takes honey in milk, he becomes energetic and disease free.
2. It makes human body healthy, beautiful and glowing.
3. It brings youth in old age.
4. Honey reduces level of cholesterol in blood.
5. It increases resistance power.
6. Honey removes weakness of respiratory system, nervous system and ailments relating to skin.
7. Consuming honey is very beneficial in problems of digestive system.
8. It also has antiseptic qualities.
9. If children are given honey mixed with milk before sleeping then the bed-wetting problem is cured.
10. Giving mixture of honey and banana to a child, cures his habit of eating mud.
11. Giving one portion honey with 2 portions of curd to children kills the germs of the stomach.
12. Giving honey to a child during teething will reduce his agony and keep him healthy.
13. It is beneficial in both high and low BP.
14. Taking one spoon honey before sleeping, stops the problem of frequent urination.

Honey

Note – Honey and water mixture should always be taken on empty stomach. Mixing honey in very hot water is harmful. During winters, luke warm water should be added. Honey should never be heated on flame.

Detection of Pure Honey

1. Pure honey has fragrance. It sets in winters and melts in summer.
2. Pure honey does not leave spot when put on paper and cloth.
3. It is transparent to look at. A dog will smell it and leave it, he will not have it.
4. Pure honey when dropped in a plate, drops like a snake curling, whereas impure honey spreads on dropping.
5. When we put pure honey on a bee it does not die but comes out.
6. Soak a piece of cotton in honey. Then burn it. If the honey is pure then the cotton will easily burn but if sugar is mixed in honey, it will not burn. Even if it burns there will be crackling sound.
7. Whether the honey is pure or impure to find out, put a single drop in water, if it dissolves it is impure, if it does not it is pure.
8. To test the purity of honey through laboratory test, heat approximately 10 grams honey with Sodium Bisulphate and Barium, if it sets, then jaggery is mixed in honey.

High Quality Nutrition in Seeds and Nuts

Seeds have complete protein, carbohydrate, fat (unsaturated), natural salts, vitamins, lecithin, etc., which are necessary for us.

In summers the cold beverage of cucumber, bottle gourd, water-melon and pumpkin seeds is very beneficial.

Milk of sunflower seed is the store house of vitamin-D. It increases masculine strength. It is a complete food and has lot of minerals.

Among these flax, sesame and groundnut have been given special importance.

Flax Seed

It is used as food and as well as a medicine. It has vitamin-F in abundance. It is full of lecithin.

It is source of necessary omega-3 fatty acid which is very important for the heart. It is very beneficial in poly-cystic ovary. It's powder can be consumed by mixing in vegetables or flour. It's oil is also used for eating.

Sesame

Consuming sesame brings almost magical strength in a human being, that he can fulfil his firm aims.

Eating it in winters is of special importance. During winters eating it, especially in Magha (January-February) is a custom.

Following are the reasons for sesame and its products being of high quality –

1. It is a source of vitamins E, B, C and F.

2. It is a good source of required calcium and phosphorus for teeth and bones and iron for blood.
3. It has high quality of protein and all necessary amino acid. It neither causes constipation nor forms gases. Being full of alkaline constituents it stops the acidic effect of protein.
4. Nature has made it a nutritious treasure, therefore its usage provides all necessary elements.
5. As compared to acidic and cholesterol rich fats this is much better.
6. It is a good source of lecithin.

Groundnut

For the common man, nature has provided the easily available food, groundnut in comparison to almond. From the view of nutrition, groundnut has almost same elements as that of almond.

Groundnut has useful protein and necessary amino acid in abundance. 100 gram groundnut has same protein as in 1 litre of milk.

Groundnut has unsaturated fat. It is the best source of calcium, phosphorus and iron.

Various vitamins are found in it in good quality.

Groundnut is very nutritious for women during pregnancy and breast feeding period.

Raw groundnut should be consumed after being soaked or sprouted. It is very beneficial for heart patients and diabetics. It improves memory.

Milk is also prepared from groundnut.

Coconut

Due to its qualities, coconut is considered as a sacred fruit in Indian culture and in almost all the Indian festivals, coconut is used. The usefulness of coconut is mentioned in various places in the Vedas and other religious books.

Coconut works both as a food and as a medicine. It has vitamins A, B, C and minerals calcium, iron, phosphorus minerals in sufficient quantity. It has high quality alkaline oil by which the body gets adequate fats. The protein found in it is of high quality and its carbohydrate enhances growth.

Coconut is cooling, easily digestible, nutritious, energy giver and improves blood and enzymes, urinary cleansing and removes Vata, Pitta and blood toxins. Its dry nut is oily, full of taste and enhances energy.

Chewing coconut daily, avoids all types of mouth cancer. If pregnant lady consumes coconut then the child born is healthy and strong and delivery will not be too painful and constipation is also removed. It works as an antioxidant.

Coconut milk is very beneficial for stomach ulcer, constipation, colitis and for people with weak digestion power.

Eating coconut increases the vigour of body and beauty is enhanced and it keeps the heart pure.

Soya Bean

It is difficult to find any other food in the world which is as nutritious as soya bean. The place of soya bean is not less than milk in any way. Protein of soya bean is much more useful and better than that of almond, milk and meat. It is a source of calcium and phosphorus and has vitamins in abundance. Its fat has an element called lecithin which reduces cholesterol, hence beneficial for heart patients.

Soya bean is healthy and energy enhancer. Lungs become strong on consuming soya bean. Its consumption removes weakness of brain. On consuming soya bean, the skin becomes soft and oily and starts glowing. Nails become pinkish.

It is especially useful in anaemia.

It keeps the nerves relaxed and removes irritability. It has such elements which can repair the brain. It is especially useful for pregnant and breast feeding woman.

Ways of Consumption

1) Mix 10% soya bean flour in wheat flour for making chapatis.
2) Make curries by mixing in whole grain, gram, rajma and chole.
3) Making curries of only soya bean.
4) Soaking and sprouting soya bean.
5) Making milk, curd or cheese of soya bean.

Milk

Mother's milk is the best quality food for a child. He requires this milk till the tooth appears and the working capacity of digestive organs is completed. Beyond that, all his requirements are met by balanced food. Then he does not require milk.

Nature provides new born children with lactase enzyme which helps in digestion of lactose or milk sugar. This capacity ends till the child reaches the age of 4 or 5 years. Lactose is comparatively such a big element, which the blood flow is not able to absorb unless it is divided into galactose and glucose and for this purpose, lactase is supposed to be very necessary.

Most people take milk after dinner and before going to sleep. Due to this the food does not get digested. Milk should not be taken after dinner. It can be taken in the morning during breakfast.

Today getting pure milk has become very difficult.

Pasteurized Milk

Many enzymes end vitamins are destroyed by the high temperature and its protein and calcium becomes so hard that it is difficult to digest them.

Artificial Milk

After taking out the cream, refined is mixed in remaining sprata milk for greasiness. White lead is added for colour. Shampoo/detergent is mixed for lather. Ararot (Rie flour) makes the milk thick and more cream extract out. Hydrogen is mixed to keep it fresh for long time. Regular consumption of artificial milk leads heart disease, liver problem, cancer and other severe diseases.

Synthetic Milk

Many harmful chemicals such as caustic soda, urea, blotting paper, hydrogen peroxide, formalin, etc., are mixed for making synthetic milk. Synthetic sugar is added to increase sweetness. This leads to many diseases such as ulcer, skin disease, mental problem and cancer. The level of disease will depend on the amount of chemicals and the time since they are being consumed. The effect of this does not show immediately, but once they start, it gets difficult to control them.

Ill effect of Oxytocin injection on milk

These days people in milk business are using much of oxytocin injection on animals. Due to the effect of injections, harmful elements from the animal's body get mixed into the milk which are harmful for human health and by drinking this a person's mental balance gets disturbed. Easy occurrence of anger and aggression are its example. It has ill-effect on endocrine glands of a person and as a result, dangerous diseases like paralysis and cancer occur. Oxytocin injection also adversely affects the reproductive power of human beings.

The capacity to hear and vision decreases, one gets easily tired, girls have early puberty, abnormal growth, miscarriage and less production of milk, etc.

Alternatives of Milk (Natural Milk)

Milk of soya bean, sesame, groundnut, coconut, dry fruits and seeds are alternatives. For sweetening, use honey, dates or raisins.

1. Groundnut Milk

Soak raw groundnut in water for 12 hours. Grind soaked groundnut in mixer and make a paste. Strain this after adding eight to ten times warm or cold water as required and milk is ready. The consistency can be changed by changing the amount of water.

Uses – It has sufficient protein, carbohydrate, fat, vitamin-A, B, Calcium, iron and phosphorus. It is easily digestible, energetic and removes weakness of brain.

2. Sesame Milk

Soak white sesame in water for 12 hours. Grind soaked sesame in mixer and prepare a paste. Now add eight times hot or cold water as per requirement and strain it. Consistency can be changed by changing the amount of water added.

Uses – It is a store house of calcium. It has protein, carbohydrate, vitamins B, C, E, phosphorus, iron, etc., in abundance. Nature has stored treasures of known and unknown nutrients in this. Hence we get all necessary elements from it. Its fat is free of cholesterol.

It is very beneficial for nervous weakness, weakness of teeth, menstrual problem, skin problem and for increasing vital power. It is destroyer of Vata, Pitta and Kapha. Its milk can be used to make curd and cheese.

3. Coconut Milk

First Method – Grind raw coconut in mixer and make a paste. Now add eight times hot or cold water as required and strain it. Amount of water can be changed to change the consistency of milk.

Second Method – Soak dry coconut in water for 12 hours. Grind soaked coconut and make a paste. Add eight times hot or cold water as required, boil it and strain it. Amount of water can be changed to change the consistency of milk.

Uses – It has sufficient vitamins A, B, C and minerals calcium, iron, phosphorus etc. It has high quality alkaline oil and easily digestible protein and carbohydrate. It is good for health. Its usage removes constipation and all types of intestinal swelling. Children don't have rickets problem.

4. Almond Milk

Soak almond nut for 12 hours, peel it off and grind in a mixer to make a paste. Now add eight times hot or cold water as

Milk

required and strain it. The consistency can be changed by changing the amount of water.

Uses – It is specially beneficial for students and people who do mental work.

5. Cashewnut Milk

Soak cashewnut in water for 6 hours, grind it and make paste. Now add eight times hot or cold water as required and strain it. To change the consistency, change the amount of water added.

Uses – It is rich in protein. It is also beneficial for diabetics.

6. Watermelon Seed Milk

Soak watermelon seed in water for half an hour and make paste by grinding it. Now add six times water to it and strain it. The milk is ready.

Uses – It has calcium and phosphorus in abundance. It keeps the mind fresh.

7. Soya bean Milk

First Method – Grind dry soya bean into powder form. Boil one litre water and 100 gm soya bean powder using a spoon, put little at a time and keep stirring. In ten minutes the milk will be ready. To change the consistency of milk, change the amount of powder mixed. Cool it and add required amount of cardamom and honey.

Second Method – To make 1 litre milk, soak 100 gm soya bean in water overnight. In the morning soaked soya bean will weight 200 gm. Grind in a mixer and make a paste. Add 800 ml water, mix it properly and strain through a thick cloth. Now boil it on a low flame for 10-15 minutes and keep stirring. Cool it and add required cardamom and honey.

Uses – Soyabean milk is just as beneficial as cow's milk. In the world it is difficult to get something as nutritious as soya bean.

It is a store-house of protein and its protein is of very high quality.

It is 80% alkaline. It is a good source of calcium, iron, phosphorus and vitamin B.

Soya bean milk is always beneficial for children. It reduces cholesterol. Therefore it is very useful for heart patients and high BP. It does not produce uric acid hence is a good substitute of milk for gout patients. It improves vital power.

It is beneficial in mental problems, nervous weakness, memory loss, epilepsy, hysteria, lung diseases (especially tuberculosis), pimples, boils, pigmentation, diabetes, anaemia, liver problem, gas disorder and kidney disease, etc.

It is beneficial in all diseases of increased acidity and it also reduces the chances of cancer.

Curd and cheese can be made from this milk.

8. *Sunflower Seed's Milk*

Soak sunflower seeds in water for 12 hours and grind it to a paste in a mixer. Now add six times water and strain it. The milk is ready.

Uses – It is full of Vitamin-D. Improves masculine power. It is especially beneficial for bones.

9. *Dry Fruits Milk*

Sesame soaked for 12 hours, raw coconut, almond soaked for 12 hours and peeled, mixed in equal quantity and made a paste by grinding in a mixer. Add eight times hot or cold water as required and strain. Take it by adding honey or jaggery.

Uses – It is beneficial for improving weight, energy and masculine power.

(Similarly other nuts and seeds can be used to make natural milk)

Curd

Curd digests more quickly than milk. Those who cannot take milk due to lactose intolerance can take curd. The helpful bacteria in curd, convert the lactose of milk to lactic acid. These are very helpful in keeping our intestines healthy.

Regular consumption of curd keeps the wall of intestines healthy and strong. Consuming curd also removes many serious diseases or decreases them. Liver, kidney and heart patients have been seen to become healthy by its usage. It cures cough and gas also. It has an important role in diarrhoea and urinary discharge.

Consumption of curd strengthens our teeth and bones because it has ample calcium. It is the best food to keep digestive power properly active. It strengthens the digestive system.

Curd has the power to reduce cholesterol. Therefore it has been proved to be a bliss for heart patients. Not only this, it is also useful for high BP and kidney patients. If anyone suffers from insomnia, then he must definitely consume curd. One gets good sleep after taking curd.

Excessive usage of antibiotics damage the helpful bacteria (probiotic) of digestive system and destroy them. By eating curd the helpful bacteria gets developed and the person again starts getting vitality and youth. Curd not only has the capacity to stop cancer but is also a natural antibiotic. Consumption of curd is good in diabetes. *Note* –
1. Curd should not be consumed at night.
2. Curd should always be beaten properly before eating.
3. Sour curd should not be consumed as it is harmful for health.

If the curd has turned sour then hang it in a thin cloth and when the water is removed add raw milk and beat it.

If the milk has turned very sour then add 3 times water to it. After 45 minutes remove all the water of the top. The sourness of curd will be removed.

To settle the curd fast, heat the milk slightly. Now add little curd and mix it 2-3 times by pouring in another container, then keep it in a casserole. The curd will set quickly.

Sometimes the curd does not settle, in such cases heat water in a container with big opening. Now without moving, keep the container with unsettled curd in this. After half an hour the settled curd will be ready.

To settle the curd easily during winters, keep the container of curd in a pressure cooker filled with hot water or casserole.

To settle the curd easily and quickly during winters, also warm milk in a container, add one teaspoon curd and keep the container in flour box by covering it. The curd will be ready in about 6 hours.

To make the curd firm use a container made of mud.

To make firm curd, apply alum inside the container and settle the curd.

To make firm curd add one teaspoon curd to hot milk, keep this container in flour or rice box by covering it. In about 6 hours the curd will be ready.

The use of chemicals in preparation of milk has put a question mark on the purity of milk. Therefore it is better to prepare curd from, milk of soya bean, groundnut or dry fruits.

Various Uncooked Preparations

Nature has already given various types of fruits, leaves, vegetables, liquid natural drinks, dry fruits, seeds and grains in the form of uncooked food.

Every food made by nature has complete natural ease, beauty, sweetness, fragrance and taste but man does not accept this easily. In haughtiness of being intelligent and knowledgeable or in innocence, he breaks the ease of his food, mixes one fragrance with another, destroys the taste of two three things and creates a new taste, changes the natural look and colour of every thing and gives the look and shape of his own choice.

Therefore through various dishes (chutney, raita, drinks/ beverages, mixed salad, sprout salad, sweets, etc.) of uncooked food new taste and look can be obtained and uncooked food can be easily adopted in life.

In dishes of uncooked food, red chillies, garam masala, white sugar, ghee, etc., shall not be used. For sweetness, jaggery (without masala), powder of dry dates or honey can be used.

In some dishes roasting is used so that the dish can be made properly. But this is not in accordance with uncooked food but still is better for all who do not adopt 100% uncooked food.

Chutneys

Chutney is easily digestible and good food for those who have weak digestion.

Mixing coconut, groundnut, sesame, cashewnut, sprouted grains, etc., to chutney and taking them in required amount works like a complete balanced food.

Protein and fat has good combination with green leafy vegetables thus a mixture of these in chutney is a food of good combination. Keeping chutneys for a long time (even in the fridge) destroys its benefits. Therefore chutney should be prepared only when all the other dishes are ready.

To make the chutney sour any one element like lemon, tamarind, amla, pomegranate seeds, curd, etc., can be used.

Some examples are illustrated below. Apart from them, various other types of chutneys with various combinations can be made according to taste.

1. Mint Chutney

Ingredients :

Mint	– 25 gm (1 cup)
Green chilly (small)	– 1
Ginger	– 1 (small piece)
Lemon juice, raw mango or tamarind etc.	– as per taste.

Method : cut everything and grind together.

2. Sweet Mint Chutney

Ingredients :

Green Mint	– 25 gm (1 cup)
Green coriander	– 50 gm (2 cup)
Ginger (finely grated)	– 1 tea-spoon
Green chilly (small)	– 2

For sweetness add soaked dates (8) or soaked black raisin (15) or powder of jaggery 2 big spoons as required.

Method : Add lemon, cumin as per taste and make chutney.

3. Tomato Chutney (Sauce)

Ingredients :

Tomato (cut into small pieces)	– 300 gm (2 cup)
Onion (cut into small pieces)	– 150 gm (1 cup)
Dates	– 10 piece
Cumin, ginger	– as per taste

Method : Mix all the ingredients in mixer and make chutney. Add water as per the requirement.

Various Uncooked Preparations 71

4. Onion Chutney

Ingredients :
Onion (finely grated)	– 150 gm (1 cup)
Ginger (finely grated)	– 1 tea-spoon
Ground cumin and green chilly	– as per taste
Green coriander (cut finely)	– 50 gm (2 cup)
Lemon	– half

Method : Grind all ingredients and add lemon juice.

5. Green Coconut Chutney

Ingredients :
Coriander	– 50 gm (2 cup)
Mint	– 25 gm (1 cup)
Fresh coconut (grated)	– 75 gm (1 cup)
Ginger, cumin, green chilly and lemon	– as per taste.

Method : Mix all ingredients and grind into chutney. Note : Garlic can also be added.

6. Sweet Coconut Chutney

Ingredients :
Raw coconut (grated)	– 75 gm (1 cup)
Dates	– 8 pieces
Pepper	– 6
Cardamom	– 3

Method : Grind all the above and make a chutney. Note : This chutney is very beneficial, nutritious and destroys constipation when used with fruits.

7. Coconut Sesame Chutney

Ingredients :
Raw coconut (grated)	– 150 gm (2 cup)
Black sesame soaked	– 25 gm (3 tea-spoon)
White sesame soaked	– 50 gm (6 tea-spoon)
Curry leaves	– 10 gm
Pepper	– 10 pieces

Method : Grind all ingredients to a chutney.
Note : This is very good for removing calcium deficiency from the body.

8. Coconut-Gram Chutney

Ingredients :

Coconut (grated)	– 150 gm (2 cup)
Roasted gram	– 25 gm (3 spoon)
Green coriander	– 25 gm (1 cup)
Green chilly	– 1
Lemon juice	– 2 tea-spoon
Ginger	– 1 small piece

(Garlic can be added if desired).
Method : Grind the ingredients and add lemon juice.

9. Coconut groundnut chutney

Ingredients :

Coriander	– 50 gm (2 cup)
Mint	– 12 gm (1/2 cup)
Fresh coconut (grated)	– 1 cup
Groundnut pieces (soaked)	– 1 cup
Date	– 6 pieces
Tamarind juice	– 2 tea-spoon
Ginger, cumin, green chilly	– as per taste
Garlic (optional)	– 2 flakes

Method : Except coriander and mint, grind all other ingredients coarsely, now add coriander and mint and grind into chutney. If required, add little water.

10. Groundnut Chutney

Ingredients :

Soaked Groundnut	– 50 gm
Green coriander	– 1 cup
Ginger	– 1 small piece
Lemon	– half
Garlic (optional)	– 2 flakes

Method : Grind all and mix lemon juice.

Various Uncooked Preparations

11. Special Chutney

Ingredients :

Coconut	– 50 gm
Raw soaked groundnut	– 50 gm
White sesame (soaked)	– 50 gm
Coriander leaves	– 50 gm

Lemon can be added for taste.
Method : Grind all and make a chutney.

12. Sweet 'n' Sour Chutney

Ingredients :

Dates (cleaned)	– 100 gm (1 cup)
Tamarind (cleaned)	– 50 gm (half cup)
Cumin (ground)	– 1 tea spoon

Method : Soak dates and tamarind in water for 2-3 hours and after they become soft grind it in the mixer or by hand and sieve it through a thin sieve and mix cumin powder.
Note–Pieces of ripe banana can be mixed in it.

13. Amla Chutney

Ingredients :

Green amla	– 2
Green coriander	– 25 gm
Cumin	– 1/2 tea spoon
Dates	– 2
Garlic (optional)	– 2 flakes

Method : Cut the amla finely, add rest of the ingredients and make a chutney.

14. Cough Repressive Chutney

Ingredients :

Flax seeds	– 50 gm
Garlic	– 25 gm
Coconut	– 50 gm
Turmeric	– little

Method : Grind all and make a chutney.
Other Method : Instead of flax seeds, black or white sesame can be used.

Drinks

The good and useful elements of fruits and vegetables is obtained in form of juices. Apart from being naturally alkaline and storehouse of water soluble minerals, juices have another advantage, that they can be consumed in more quantity as compared to fruits and vegetables.

Innumerable tasty drinks can be prepared from this necessary group of food substances.

1. Carrot Drink

Ingredients :

Carrot juice	– 4 cup
Coconut milk	– 1 cup
Dates (soaked for sometime)	– 3 or 4

Method : Mix in a mixer properly. Strain and use.

2. Pink Milk

Ingredients :

Coconut or cow's milk	– 2 cup
Normal cold water	– 4 cup
Rose water	– half cup
Honey or other sweetener	– as per liking
Beetroot juice	– 2 tea-spoon

Method : Mix all ingredients in a bowl. Beetroot will give pink colour.

3. Cucumber Drink

Ingredients :

Cucumber	– 200 gm
Tomato	– 100 gm
Green coriander	– 25 gm
Mint	– 25 gm
Ginger	– 1 small piece
Lemon	– as per taste

Method : Except lemon, extract juice of all other ingredients in a juicer and then mix lemon juice.

Various Uncooked Preparations

4. Spinach Drink

Ingredients :

Spinach juice	– 3 cup
Coconut milk	– 1 cup
Honey	– as per taste

Method : Make by adding water as required.

5. Tomato Drink

Ingredients :

Ripe red tomatoes	– 400 gm
Soaked cashewnuts	– 8-10
Coriander, mint	– 100 gm
Ginger	– 1 small piece
Cumin	– as per taste
Honey or dates	– as required

Method : Put ingredients in mixer and extract the juice. Strain and add honey.

6. Papaya Shake

Ingredients :

Ripe papaya	– 200 gm
Honey	– 1 big spoon
Ripe banana	– 50 gm
Ground cardamom	– 1 pinch

Method : Mix papaya and banana in a mixer by adding little water. Now add honey and ground cardamom.

7. Thandai

Ingredients :

Seeds of watermelon and melon (soaked for 4-5 hours)	– 2 Table spoon
Dates	– 5
Aniseed	– 1 tea-spoon
Rose petals	– 1 tea-spoon
Poppy seeds	– 1 tea-spoon
Pepper	– 4-6 pieces

Method : Put all the ingredients in a mixer and grind it finely. Strain and drink.

Other Method : In the same way coconut, almond and sesame thandai can also be made.

8. Various type of drinks

In various fruit juices, sugarcane juice, coconut water, etc., or any sour substance like lemon, tamarind or amla can be added or honey and any other sweetener can be added to make various types of drinks.

Raita

Everybody knows to make raita in curd but most people add boiled or squeezed cucumber and bottlegourd, by which they destroy the nutrient values. Cucumber, vegetable marrow, bottlegourd, etc., should always be grated raw and leafy vegetables like spinach, mint, white goose poot should be used after making a paste.

1. Tomato Raita

Ingredients :

Tomato	– 500 gm
Thick Curd	– 400 gm
Green coriander	– 50 gm

Method : Finely cut tomatoes and green coriander and mix in curd.

Other Method : In the same way bottle gourd, cucumber, carrot, onion, etc., can be grated and made into raita.

2. Mint Raita

Ingredients :

Mint	– 100 gm
Curd	– 400 gm

Method : Make fine paste of mint leaves in a mixer and add to curd. Dry mint can also be used.

Other Method : Similarly raita can be made of white goose poot (Bathua), spinach, etc.

In the same way various type of raitas can be made.

Various Uncooked Preparations

Sprouted Salad

Sprouted grains can be mixed with different food substances to make new, tasty and attractive dishes.

1. Sprouted Wheat Salad

Ingredients :
Sprouted wheat	– 100 gm
Small piece of raisin or dates	– 20 gm
Green coriander	– little

Method : Mix all the ingredients.
Other Method : Sprouted alfalfa can also be added to this.

2. Sprouted Green Gram (Moong) Salad

Ingredients :
Sprouted green gram	– 25 gm
Cabbage	– 25 gm
Carrot	– 50 gm
Green coriander and lemon juice	– as per taste

Method : (1) Cut pieces of carrot and cabbage and mix in sprouted moong.
(2) Add lemon juice and green coriander to this mixture.

Note : Instead of sprouted green gram, sprouted moth can be used or even both can be used. Other Method : In the same way, other seasonal vegetables like tomato, onion, beetroot, etc., can be used to create various new tastes.

3. Mixed Sprouted Salad

Ingredients :
Sprouted green gram, moth	– 250 gm
Sprouted grain	– 50 gm
Soaked groundnut	– 100 gm
Small pieces of raisin or dates	– 50 gm
Raw coconut (grated)	– 50 gm
Green coriander	– as required

Method : Mix all of them together.
Other Method : Sprouted alfalfa, soaked dry fruits, tomato, cucumber, etc., can be added and new mixtures to be made of different taste and look.

4. Sprouted Alfalfa Salad

Ingredients :

Sprouted alfalfa	– 100 gm
Small pieces of tomato	– 50 gm
Carrot or cucumber (grated)	– 50 gm
Green coriander	– little
Lemon	– as per taste

Method : Mix all of them and add lemon juice.

Mixed Salad

Various types of vitamins, minerals and nutritious fibrous food is obtained from salad. To make salad, it is necessary for the vegetables to be fresh. Of these vegetable, the most important is salad leaves. For salad, radish, carrot, tomato, cucumber, cabbage and capsicum are useful things. Various mixtures can be made and complete pleasure can be obtained from new salad dishes.

Salad No. 1

Ingredients :

Onion	– 25 gm
Tomato	– 10 gm
Carrot	– 100 gm
Cucumber	– 100 gm
Cabbage leaves	– 50 gm
Mint leaves (chopped)	– 1/2 spoon
Pepper	– 1/4 spoon

Method : Cut all the ingredients and add lemon and pepper.

Salad No. 2

Ingredients :

Finely chopped cabbage	– 2 cup
Spinach and radish leaves (finely chopped)	– 1 cup
Pieces of tomato	– 1 cup
Green coriander	– as per taste.

Method : Mix all.

Various Uncooked Preparations

Salad No. 3

Ingredients :
Green fenugreek leaves	– 25 gm
Carrot	– 25 gm
Cucumber	– 30 gm
Onion (optional)	– 25 gm
Lemon juice	– as per taste

Method : Cut all the vegetables and add lemon juice.

Salad No. 4

Ingredients :
Finely grated cauliflower	– 3 cup
Grated carrot	– 1 cup
Grated beetroot	– 1/2 cup
Tomato pieces	– 1/2 cup
Finely cut spinach	– 1 cup
Green coriander	– as required.

Method : Mix them all.

Salad No. 5

Ingredients :
Finely cut cabbage	– 2 cup
Fenugreek leaves or white goose poot	– 1 cup
Finely cut coriander and mint	– 1/2 cup
Lemon, green chilly	– as per taste
Onion (optional)	– 1/2 cup

Method : Mix them all.

Salad No. 6

Ingredients :
Big tomatoes	– 2
Grated beetroot	– 1 cup

Method : Add tomato pieces to grated beetroot.

Salad No. 7

Ingredients :
Finely grated carrot	– 2 cup
Grated raw coconut	– 1 cup
Lemon	– 1

Method : Squeeze lemon juice and add all.

Salad No. 8

Ingredients :
Finely cut cabbage	– 2 cup
Peas	– 3/4 cup
Tomatoes	– 3/4 cup
Grated coconut	– 1/2 cup

Method : Mix all.

Salad No. 9

Ingredients :
Small pieces of vegetable marrow or cucumber	– 2 cup
Small pieces of tomato	– 1 cup
Finely cut onion	– 1/2 cup
Coriander, mint and green chilly	– as per taste

Method : Add them all.

Salad No. 10

Ingredients :
Finely cut cabbage	– 2 cup
Finely grated carrot	– 1 cup
Capsicum/cut into thin small pieces	– 1/2 cup
Lemon	– 1

Method : Mix all and add juice of full 1 lemon.

Salad No. 11

Ingredients :
Finely grated cabbage	– 1 cup
Finely grated coconut	– 1/2 cup
Finely cut onion	– 1/2 cup
Finely grated carrot	– 3/4 cup

Green spices–Coriander, mint, lemon, ginger, fresh turmeric, amla, turmeric, green chilly, etc., as per taste.

Method : Mix all the things. Garnish with coconut and coriander and serve.

Various Uncooked Preparations 81

Salad No. 12

Ingredients :

Tomato	– 100 gm
Cucumber	– 120 gm
Cauliflower	– 100 gm
Sweet Corn	– 4 tea-spoon
Lemon juice	– 1 tea-spoon

Method : Cut tomato, cucumber, cauliflower into small pieces, add sweet corn and lemon juice.

Salad No. 13

Ingredients :

Finely cut cabbage	– 2 cup
Medium sized red, ripe tomatoes	– 4
Honey	– 4 tea-spoon
Finely grated coconut	– 1 cup

Method : Cut round or semi circular slices of tomatoes and decorate in a big plate. On top of it make 1st layer of finely cut cabbage and 2nd layer of coconut. Put little honey on each tomato. In place of honey, juice of raisin or dates can also be used.

Note : Decoration of cashewnut, walnut or almond will increase its nutrition and work as a complete balanced food.

Salad No. 14

Ingredients :

Carrot (grated)	– 550 gm
Beetroot (grated)	– 50 gm
Turnip (grated)	– 15 gm
Radish (grated)	– 30 gm
Parsley (chopped)	– 15 gm
Tomato (sliced)	– 50 gm
Ajwain leaves (chopped)	– 10 gm
Cabbage leaves (chopped)	– 20 gm
Cucumber (Sliced)	– 50 gm
Ground coriander	– 1/2 tea-spoon
Ground cumin	– 1/2 tea-spoon
Lemon juice	– as required.

Method : Mix all the ingredients and add ground coriander, ground cumin and lemon juice.

Sweets

Sweets is always everybody's favourite. We buy different sweets from the market. There is no guarantee of its purity and moreover instead of being nutritious they are harmful for health. Why not make, eat and serve such sweets which are pure, nutritious and interesting- the one which does not have oil, ghee or sugar and which does not require frying or cooking.

1. Sesame and Dates Comfit (Laddoo)

Ingredients :
White sesame	– 40%
Dates	– 60%

Cut the dates after removing the seeds. Roast the white sesame lightly in a pan. Grind the sesame while it is hot. Now mix the dates and grind them again. Take out the mixture and make laddoos.

Other Method : In the same way cashewnut or groundnut can be used instead of sesame.

2. Sesame, dryfruits and dates comfit (laddoo)

Ingredients :
Sesame	– 200 gm
Dates	– 500 gm
Poppy seeds	– 50 gm
Almond or cashew nut	– 50 gm

Method : Cut the dates after removing the seeds. Roast the white sesame lightly in a pan. While the sesame is hot add dates, powdered poppy seeds and almonds or cashewnut and grind again. Take out the mixture and make laddoos.

3. Coconut and Cashewnut sweet (Burfi)

Ingredients :
Dry coconut finely grated	– 3 cup
Cashewnut	– 1 cup

Various Uncooked Preparations

Honey	– 1/2 cup or as per taste
Cardamom (ground)	– 1 tea spoon
Rose water	– 1/2 cup
Piyal seeds	– 1 table spoon

Method : Finely grind dry coconut and cashewnut separately in a mixer. Take both the powder in a big plate, add honey, rose water, cardamom and knead it. Spread it in a plate and set it like burfi. Garnish with piyal seeds.

4. Coconut raisin sweet (Burfi)

Ingredients :

Raisin	– 1 cup
Grated dry coconut	– 1 cup
Cardamom powder	– 2 tea spoon
Payal seeds or cashew nuts	– As required

Method : Grind dry coconut and raisin finely in a mixer. Take it out on a plate and mix cardamom powder. Spread it in a big plate by making a thick layer for Burfi. Garnish it with chironji and cashewnut pieces. Cut like burfi and use.

Other Method : Fresh coconut can be used in place of dry coconut.

5. Carrot Comfit (Laddoo)

Ingredients :

Finely grated carrot	– 2 cup
Finely grated coconut	– 1 cup
Finely cut dates	– 3 cup
Cardamom powder	– 1 tea spoon

Method : Mix carrot, dates and cardamom and make its laddoos. Roll it in grated coconut and use them while fresh.

6. Cashewnut and coconut Pedas

Ingredients :

Cashewnut	– 1 cup
Grated dry coconut	– 1 cup
Cardamom powder	– 1/2 spoon
Honey	– 2 table spoon

Method: Grind cashewnut and dry coconut to a powder form, take it in a plate, add honey and cardamom and mix it. Make in shape of pedas.

7. Stuffed Dates

Ingredients:
Dates	– 100 gm
Cashewnut powder	– 50 gm
Cardamom	– as per taste

Method: Remove the seeds from dates and cut into half. Mix cashewnut powder and cardamom. Fill this mixture in half piece of date. Press with hand and give attractive shape and look.
Other Method: Similarly instead of cashewnut powder, walnut powder, coconut, almond, groundnut, sesame, melon and water melon seed, poppy seed, etc., can be used. Among these various mixed powder can also be used. In this way many sweets can be made.

8. Wheat bran porridge (Halwa)

Ingredients:
Jaggery	– 100 gm
Wheat bran	– 100 gm
Ghee	– little

Method: Take jaggery in a pan and heat it in a pan on low flame. Add wheat bran and mix. Remove and apply little ghee. Halwa is ready.

9. Wheat bran comfit (Laddoo)

Ingredients:
Dates	– 100 gm
Wheat bran	– 100 gm

Method: Remove the seed of dates and grind along with wheat bran in a mixer. Make laddoo from the mixture.
Secret of Health Uncooked Food

10. Special Comfit (Laddoo)

Ingredients:
Dates	– 5 kgs.
Roasted groundnut	– 500 gm

Various Uncooked Preparations 85

Sesame	– 500 gm
Dry coconut	– 500 gm
Cashewnut	– 500 gm
Watermelon seeds	– 500 gm
Almond	– 500 gm
Cardamom	– 50 gm

Method : Rub the dates with cloth and remove the seed. Roast the sesame in a pan and grind it. While it is hot, add powder of remaining ingredients and dates and make a mixture. Make laddoos from this mixture. These can also be taken while travelling.

11. Fruit Cream

Ingredients :

Cream of milk	– 200 gm
Various type of fruits	– 500 gm

Method : Cut all types of available fruits in small pieces and mix them in cream. Note : Raisin or dates pieces can also be added to this.

MEASURES AND WEIGHTS

1 Tea-spoon full (TSF) = 5 gm or 5 ml.
1 Cup or 1/2 Glass = 125 ml.

Think

that use of artificial drinks, fried and cooked unnatural food, sweets, tea, coffee and alcohol, etc., during festivals, picnics and parties are sowing the seed of diseases in us, relatives and guests. Our festivals can be celebrated with fruits, juices, natural sweets and simple cooked food which improve health and double our pleasure.

Food of Special Quality

Basil (Tulsi)

Basil has not only religious importance, but it has a unique place due to its medicinal benefits. Basil odour mixed with air keeps the environment healthy and stops the growth of harmful insects like mosquitoes, flies, etc. Mainly, basil is of two types—
1. Shyam basil (black stem and black leaves)
2. Ram basil (white stem and green leaves).

Both the basils are approximately same in properties and odour. Yet Shyam basil is considered to be of a better quality than Ram basil. A man eating five leaves of basil a day is safe against many types of diseases. It cures mental weakness and increases mental and memory power. Aged persons using basil daily never feel weakness and are safe against communicable (infectious) diseases. Leaves of basil are a blood purifier. Its use automatically increases beauty (glow). The disease curing property of basil makes it a panacea. Today human beings can be cured easily from all diseases by the use of basil only.

In Ayurveda, basil is called 'Tridosh' (Vata, Pitta, and Kapha) remover.

Basil Juice—

Use of basil juice with water every morning increases the glow of the skin and memory power. It increases the digestive power. It is a worm killer. Basil's juice stops vomiting immediately. In Malaria, basil's juice is beneficial. It increases the working power of our kidney.

It is also beneficial in acidity, diarrhoea, leucoderma, and obesity. Basil's juice gives tremendous relief to patient suffering from fever, cough, cataract, cold and asthma.

Basil's juice mixed with honey should be given to the patient having internal stones, for six months.

Basil's juice decreases cholesterol in blood.

Margosa (Neem) Leaves

Margosa is a very useful tree. All its parts from root to stem, peel, flower, leaves and fruits are full of medicinal quality. Bitterness of margosa is its merit. In summer season, when all trees shed leaves, margosa is in full greenery. Some chemicals in the margosa are insect killers. Eating five soft leaves of margosa everyday cures all diseases. It purifies blood and protects from communicable diseases. It cures all dental diseases also. It makes the voice melodious. Applying margosa leaves paste on acne/boils gives tremendous relief.

During the spread of communicable diseases, eating five leaves of margosa and five leaves of basils protects us from infections.

Amla (Emblic Myrobalan)

Amla is a food as well as a medicine. It is equivalent to hundred medicines. It has a great importance in Ayurveda. In eating it, it is astringent, sweet and cool. Due to its astringent qualities, it is useful in curing Kapha and Vata and its sweetness and coolness cures Pitta. So it is a Tridosh remover. Amla is a great source of vitamin C. Its property is that vitamins in it are not destroyed on boiling and frying.

Amla gives feelings of youthfulness to both younger and aged persons. With its use, Sage Chyavan regained his youthfulness.

Amla is the only one which has properties like disease resistant, blood purifier and sperm enhancer.

So, a health cautious person should give much preference to amla in their daily diet. Amla strengthens teeth and gums

and provides activeness to the body. It is useful in nerve disorder, heart anxiety, pulsation, obesity, spleen, blood pressure, eczema, weakness in uterus, skin diseases, urine diseases and bones related diseases. For a weak liver and jaundice eradication, amla mixed with honey acts as a tonic.
Amla enhances mental power.
Its use is beneficial in arthritis.
Patients having internal stone must eat amla.
Use of amla stops hair fall and prevents them from becoming white.
Amla can be used as juice, sauce (chutney) or powder with water.

Lemon

Lemon is enriched in phosphorus, potassium, vitamin C, sulphur, folic acid, chlorine, vitamin B-1, B-6, magnesium. It is a digestive, worm killer, and remover of stomach disease. It is Tridosh (Vata, Pitta, Kapha) remover. It can be used in every season. In spite of its sourness, it is alkaline in nature.

Lemon removes extra stored waste substances or toxins from the body. Calcium, which is a key source for the formation of teeth and bones is also found in lemon. It has special properties to cure the heart's weakness. It has a lot of medical benefits so it can be used for curing different diseases. It is used for beauty. It removes obesity. Its use increases appetite and digestion. It dissolves the stone in gall bladder. It strengthens liver and kidney. It removes constipation. Having juice of a lemon in one glass of water with honey everyday with empty stomach increases body power and eye sight.

Triphala

Triphala is a mixture of one part of Harad, two part of Baheda and four parts of Amla. It is an ordinary diet food as well as a medicine. It has all the taste (bitter, sour, astringent, pungent, sweet and salty). Triphala cures the diseases and increase living power. It increases appetite. It keeps stomach clean and gives a sound sleep.

It is very beneficial to have one spoon of triphala with fresh water in the morning. Use of triphala cures sexual weakness, menstrual disorder in women and leucorrhoea.

Benefits of taking triphala upto twelve year –

Upto one year	— Overcome laziness
Upto two year	— Freedom from all disease
Upto three year	— Improvement in eye sight
Upto four year	— Increases beauty
Upto five year	— Development of intelligence
Upto six year	— Strengthens the body
Upto seven year	— Blackening of hair
Upto eight year	— Old regain youthfulness
Upto nine year	— Special power in the eyes
Upto ten year	— Improvement in voice
Upto eleven year	— Towards clairvoyance
Upto twelve year	— Clairvoyance

(For clairvoyance it is necessary to do Ashtanga Yoga).

Wheat Bran — Full of Merits

Outer layer of the wheat is known as bran or Bhusi. Usually we suffer a loss by considering this part of wheat as useless.

1/5th part of wheat weight is bran. But in this fifth part 75% of nutritious elements of wheat are present. Its chemical analysis tells that it has 12% protein and one-third starch. It is rich in calcium, iron and other minerals.

Bran provides power and activeness to the intestines. Use of bran keeps away intestinal disease. It prevents fistula and colon cancer.

It is very useful in reducing cholesterol in blood. Bran has some element which affects genes.

It removes neurological weakness; is useful in the formation of muscles and bones.

It increases haemoglobin in blood.

It is beneficial in diabetes.

It keeps the stomach clean and thus the heart and mind remain healthy. It is alkaline in nature, hence increases immunity. To reduce obesity, bran is very useful. Hence give place to bran in the diet. Mix it with flour or use it with honey. Mix it with jaggery (gur) and make small balls (Laddu). Eat it with milk or curd.

Food Combinations

To digest different elements of foods, different digestive juices are required. Starch requires alkaline digestive juice whereas protein requires acidic digestive juice. If both the foods are taken together then their digestive juice will be secreted simultaneously. Thus acidic juice and alkaline juice will neutralize each other. As a result protein starts rotting and starch (carbohydrate) starts fermenting. In the same way eating many things together like vegetables, fruits, pickles, curd, kheer, sweet and papad, etc., starts chemical reactions in the stomach and disturbs the digestive system.

One food at a time is the ideal diet. In reality, mixed food is the wrong step in itself. Less food items at a time makes the digestion easy. In a diet, fruits at one time and then salad (vegetables) at other time and then grain should be consumed. This is called mono diet.

Fruits, milk and juice should be taken separately.

Wrong Combination

1. Banana with milk or curd
2. Radish with milk or curd
3. Curd with milk
4. Hot water or other hot product with honey
5. Radish with honey
6. Sweet pudding (Kheer) with biryani (Khichdi)
7. Melon, water melon or cucumber with milk.
8. Radish with Black gram dal (Urad dal)
9. Curd with Black berry (Jamun)
10. Melon with curd
11. Cheese (Paneer) with curd

12. Vegetables with fruits
13. Curd or radish at night
14. Hot curd
15. Ghee kept in metal vessels for 10 days
16. Sweet potato, potato and kachaloo with pulses
17. Watermelon or melon with any other eatable item.
18. Pulses with rice, pulses with chapati
19. Bread with milk and curd.
20. Bread with tamarind

Note – Those who wish to have bread or rice with pulses are advised to have raw vegetables also.

Ideal combination

1. Mango and cow's milk
2. Milk and dates
3. Rice and coconut
4. Pulse and curd
5. Guava and saunf
6. Radish leaves with water melon
7. Bathua and curd (i.e. Raita)
8. Carrot and fenugreek (Methi) leaves
9. Banana and small cardamom
10. Curd with amla powder
11. Starch with leafy vegetables
12. Dry fruits with sour fruits
13. Pulses and vegetables
14. Vegetable and rice/biryani
15. Fruit and little quantity of dry fruits
16. Bread with green leafy vegetables
17. Sprouted pulses and raw coconut

Various Tastes

Appetite is a natural demand of the body. In natural appetite, every eatable item seems tasty. When there is no appetite, we need artificial tastes through pickles, jams, vinegar, salts, spices, sour, sweet etc. which is harmful to our body. It results in overeating and disturbs our digestive system.

To make food tastier, artificial colors and chemicals are being used which are harmful for the health.

Those items which cannot be eaten without salt, spices and sugar are not suitable for the body, or it is not a natural appetite.

Keep an interval of at least six hours between two meals, so that you will feel a natural appetite and every food will be tasty.

When we leave the habits of artificial tastes and adopt natural tastes, then we feel a unique pleasure which cannot be compared with any other pleasure.

The nature has gifted us different colours of fruits, leafy vegetables and dry fruits basked in sunlight with natural appeal having different tastes, fragrance, juices with full freshness, and nutrition. Each item has its own taste, e.g. different breeds of mangoes have their different taste.

Balance of Alkaline and Acidic Foods

All diseases begin from the imbalance of alkalis and acids in the body and it ends when balance is regained. The human body consists of 80 per cent alkaline elements and 20 per cent acidic elements. To remain this balance is the primary base of good health. Our physical, mental, practical, natural and vital power depends on this balance. So, our diet should consist of 80 per cent alkaline and 20 per cent acidic food.

Alkaline Foods

All types of fruits (except plum and ber), lemon, orange, leafy vegetables, green and other vegetables, coconut, fresh milk, sprouted food grains, dates, figs, soaked dry fruits, etc.

Acidic Foods

Meat, egg, cheese, butter, cooked food, chapati, dry fruits, sweets, sugar, grains, coffee, tea, chocolate, fruits in sugar syrup, boiled milk, maida, salt, tobacco, soda water, vegetable ghee, intoxicating drinks, fried items, baked products, etc.

Note – Alkaline and acidic food is not a problem for those who eat uncooked food. This is problem for only those who take cooked food.

Calcium Deficiency Filled by Uncooked Food

Calcium is important in the construction of bones, mobility of heart and muscles, to control electric power in our body, absorption of vitamins, to balance salts and to increase immune system. Vitamin D assimilates calcium in our body. Deficiency of calcium stops the growth of our bones and teeth, bones become feeble, teeth starts decaying, danger of rickets, more bleeding may happen, distortion in the heart's movements, weak nervous system, and stiffness in muscles may occur.

Causes of calcium deficiency
1. Slow absorption of calcium from food due to weak digestive system.
2. Lack of calcium substance in diet.
3. Lack of sun bath or Vitamin D
4. Lack of physical work, exercise or yoga.
5. Lack of breast feeding to infants.
6. Use of high protein diet decreases ability to get calcium in the body.
7. The possibility of calcium deficiency increases in pregnant women as the foetus gets calcium from the mother.
8. White sugar, caffeine present in tea, coffee, soft drink, etc.
9. Fast food, chocolate, acidic food, pain killer drugs, liquor, etc., excrete calcium from the body.

According to medical Director Dr. Frank A. Oski of Jones Hopkins Medical institute, protein found in animal milk excretes calcium not only from the milk but from bones through urine. This way in spite of strengthening the bone it weakens them. This is the reason because of which in Norway, Sweden and Denmark, where milk and its product are in large use, osteoporosis is also in large scale. Opposite to it is less in China, Africa where milk is not an important part of the diet.

Sources of Calcium

- In cereals — wheat, bajra, ragi, grain bran.
- In root and stem — coconut jaggery, sweet potato, yam (ratalu).
- In milk and its products — soya bean milk, sesame milk.
- In pulses — green gram dal (moong), kidney beans (rajma), lentil dal (masoor), soya bean, bengal gram (chana), moth.
- In green vegetables — curry leaves, knolkhol (Ganth gobhi) leaves, spinach, broccoli, radish leaves, fenugreek leaves, mint, green coriander.
- In other vegetables — kamal kakdi, beans, cluster beans, carrot, lady finger, tomato, cabbage, drum stick leaves, beetroot.
- In fruits — black raisin, dry date, fig, banana, papaya, orange, almond, pistachio nut, walnut.
- In seeds — melon seeds, sesame, sunflower seeds.
- In nuts — groundnuts.
- In grass — duba grass, wheat grass.

> Excess of food is always harmful.
> Each eatable should be taken in such a quantity which does not burden the stomach at that time and no heaviness is felt later on.

White Sugar — Sweet Poison

White sugar is a deformed form of natural sugar. In its digestion process many elements and vitamins get drained from the body, hampering other activities of the body.

Scientific analysis compares the sugar with liquor. It increases acidity in the body.

Excess use of sugar results in tooth decay. It is considered the root cause of arthritis. Its excessive use causes liver disease. The main cause of diabetes is also excessive use of white sugar and its product.

Excess use of it increases the possibility of cancer. It increases cholesterol in blood. It is main cause of stomach trouble. It cause sinus problems.

Mental diseases in children are due to excess use of white sugar and its product. Its excess use results in neurological weakness, menstrual pain and luecorrhoea.

To protect health, it will be good if white sugar is given up altogether. Natural sugar found in fruits and vegetables is beneficial to health as it is easily digestible. Dates, black raisins, honey and jaggery can replace sugar.

Use of Excessive Salt is Fatal

Excess salt in any substance makes it uneatable. It becomes poisonous. Similarly salt affects the inner cells, blood vessels and nerves badly. It destroys the natural taste of eatables.

Failure of kidney and liver is the result of excess salt. It affects soft parts of intestine and stomach. Its excess use results in diseases like cancer, obesity, diabetes, cold, insomnia, etc. It increases heart beat and blood pressure. It increases acidity.

Salt does not get digested easily. As the body excretes the salt by dissolving it with water, so, excess use of salt increases thirst. It works to weaken the bones as it has the ability to dissolve it.

The body gets salt from the natural substances (fruits, vegetables, sprouted grain, etc.) When eatable substances are cooked, their salt gets destroyed. So a small quantity of salt may be put in them. With natural substances (fruits, vegetables, sprout juices, curd, etc.) salt should not be used any way.

The body takes the salt from the natural eatables in an organic form. Other inorganic salts are always being excreted by the body and if they are stored in the body, it results in a severe disease. It is like a burden to our excretory organs. Salt is salt whether it is black or white.

Tea/Coffee — A Sweet Poison

Tea/Coffee has poisonous substances like tannin, caffeine, carbolic acid, oxalic acid, theine, cynogen, etc. It creates ulcers and gas in stomach. It causes dryness in the body, heaviness in the mind and lungs. The symptoms of arthritis, weakness in kidney and headache appears. The hair starts greying and there is lack of calcium in the body. Eyesight becomes weak, acidity increases, and, signs of ageing appear early. Digestive system becomes weak. Dryness appears in the intestine. Blood disorders and sexual weakness appears. Tea and coffee kills thirst, hence, due to water deficiency, poisonous substances retains in the body and results in various diseases.

Alternatives of Tea and Coffee

1. **Basil Tea** — Boil five basil leaves (dry or fresh), and taste grounded ginger, aniseed, black pepper, cardamom, etc. (according to taste) in water.
2. **Ginger Tea** — Mix a spoon of ginger juice with juice of half lemon in a glass of hot water. Drink it as a tea. It removes Vata, Pitta and Kapha.
3. **Mint Tea** — Boil 50 gm mint, 100 gm ginger, 5 gm Celery seeds in half litre of water. Mix milk and jaggery in it and drink. It removes gas and empowers digestive power.
4. **Celery seeds Tea** — Boil a half spoon of celery seeds in a cup of water, cover it for 5 minutes and add honey to it as per taste. It is beneficial in weakness of lungs.
5. **Wheat Bran Tea** — Boil 10 gm of wheat bran in a cup of water. Use it as a tea after mixing milk and jaggery. It is beneficial in catarrh, cold and headache.
6. **Wheat Bran Special Tea** — Boil 15 gm wheat bran, 10 gm ginger, 10 black pepper, 10 basil leaves, 10 black raisins

and 50 gm jaggery in half litre of water. Add milk and use. It cures old coughs, cold and anaemia.
7. **Herbal Tea** — Take boiled water and add ground basil, ginger, cardamom, aniseed, cassia leaves (Tej patta), cinnamon in same proportion. Cover it for 5 minutes. Add honey or jaggery powder after filtering it. Milk can be added. It is best for cold, cough and asthma. Patient suffering from diabetes or paralysis should also add half spoon of fenugreek seed.
8. **Special Herbal Tea** — 50 gm aniseed, 50 gm Brahmi booti, 30 gm cloves, 25 gm big cardamom, 25 gm cardamom, 30 gm Gulbanphasa, 50 gm red sandal powder, 20 gm liquorice (mulethi), 20 gm dry ginger, 10 gm black pepper, 50 gm sankhpushpi, 30 gm dry basil leaves, 15 gm cinnamon, 30 gm dry rose petals. Grind the above item separately and strain. Take 8-10 gram of above mixture and boil with half litre of water. After boiling properly, add jaggery or honey and use.

Any of the above items, whichever are available can be used as an alternative of tea.

Note — Soup of green vegetables may be used as an alternative of tea.

Spices

There is no place for spices in our daily diet. Neither our body needs them nor do they have any use to our body. These are medicines. They stimulate like medicines. Previously they were used in special diseases only. In the present day, they have become a part of our diet which is harming our body in one or another form.

It is common belief that spices increase appetite and helps digest food. Spices increase appetite as digestive juice starts excreting fast due to their pungency. Scientific analysis says that spices lack constructive nutrition. Opposite to it, they are stimulators and give burning sensations. Spices have less pros then pros.

Spices are the evidence of the fact that we are trying to consume that type of food which cannot be consumed in its typical form, but could be taken with artificial taste of spices.

Spices are medicines and can be used in diseases, if required. Frequent use of medicine is harmful. Spices are nothing more than an addiction. Only a real and true appetite can give the pleasure of eating. Spices spoil the natural taste of the food and dominate their own taste.

Due to their burning sensation, spices require us to drink more water. So, drinking water with the meal dilutes digestive enzymes which results into indigestion and diseases.

Humans are the only living things who deliberately fill poison in their body. Man destroys most of the nutrition of food by cooking it and rest of the nutrition are destroyed by adding spices. Man takes much food with the help of spices and invites several diseases by destroying digestion power.

Medicinal benefits of Spices

1. Aniseed (Saunf)

Aniseed is pungent, digestive and removes gas, fever and pain. It stops vomiting, burning sensation of urine and intestinal pain. It is liked due to its sweet taste and good fragrance. It is useful in obesity. It gives relief in indigestion, gas and constipation.

2. Asafoetida (Heeng)

In fact, this is the milk of a tree which later changes into a gum. It is has a strong odour and is black or brown in colour. It is good for appetite. It is a medicine for cough, digestive disorder and gives relief in chest pain/stomach pain. It is used in indigestion and worms diseases. It gives strength to the liver and is found effective in mental problems. It removes deposited cough from respiratory pipes (i.e. expectorant).

3. Black Pepper

Due to its pungent property, black pepper forces brain to secrets painkiller chemicals. It has property to control digestive problems. It is also useful in cough and fever.

4. Cardamom

It is one of the best things for oral fragrance. There are two types of cardamom—small and big.

Small Cardamom – It is pungent, light and cold in nature. It removes gas and cough. It is useful in respiratory diseases. It removes the bad breath. It is digestive and controls nausea.

Big Cardamom – Pungent in taste, hot, dry and light in nature. It is beneficial in cough, bile, thirst, itching, blood distortion, vomiting, mouth diseases, urinary tract problem and respiratory problems. It is also beneficial in piles.

5. Cassia/Bay leaf (Tej Patta)

It is very much beneficial in cough. It removes irregularities in menstrual periods and bath breath. It improves digestion.

6. Celery (caron) Seeds (Ajwayan)

It has a pungent smell due to a substance named thymol. It is a germ and worm killer. It serves as a good appetizer, digestive and prevents many digestive problems. It is considered beneficial for the bones as it is full of calcium. It is used for medical purposes for dysentery, gas, indigestion, stomach pain and cholera. It is also a mouth freshener.

7. Chillies

Raw chillies are green in colour and become red when ripe. It is used for giving red colour and pungent taste to the food. Red Chilli should be used in less quantity. It is better to use fresh green chilli in spite of red chilli. It stimulates the functions of the stomach.

8. Cinnamon (Dal Chini)

It is the best medicine among spices. It increases resistance power. It has a sweet fragrance. It is a good appetizer. It contains a small quantity of oil, which is a germicide and fungicide. It is a mouth freshener. It removes Tridosh (Vata, Pitta, Kapha).

9. Clove

A small black bud of clove is a mine of medicinal properties. It is bitter, pungent, light and astringent. It is kapha-pitta remover and blood purifier. It has a power to kill germs and bacteria, so it works as an antiseptic and antibiotic. It is a digestive, gas remover and appetizer. It removes pain, especially tooth pain.

Presence of Evegenol in it prevents teeth decay and stops tooth pain.

10. Coriander

Fragrance in coriander is due to a vaporizing oily substance, which is known to be a germ killer. It helps in the formation of Glutathione in our body, which helps in preventing many stomach diseases. It is pleasant, a Pitta remover and digestive.

It is beneficial in treating cough and worms in the stomach. It removes gas. It is helpful in curing mouth ulcer.

11. Cumin (Zira)

It is of two types, black and white. It is a type of an antioxidant. It is digestive and fragrant. It is found to have great effects on distaste, gas, indigestion, etc. It is a worm killer and fever preventive. It is eaten in raw form also. It is beneficial for women having less milk formation. It is also useful in stomach problem.

12. Dry Ginger

It is formed by drying ginger. It is good for the digestive system. During old age, digestive system weakens, gas formation is there and cough formation starts. For such conditions, dry ginger is the best medicine. Dry ginger is best for cough, gas and heart related diseases. It is beneficial for women after delivery.

13. Fenugreek Seeds

It is the seed of a leafy vegetable plant. It is full of medicinal properties. It keeps the sugar level down in blood. It is full of iron. Regular use of it is beneficial for anaemic patient. It is a nutritious food. It gives relief in diabetes, arthritis, constipation, gas, etc. It is an appetizer. It acts as a tonic in body pain and fatigue.

14. Ginger

Anti-bacterial elements are found in ginger. It has all the properties to increase digestion. It is a home medicine for throat problem, fever, constipation, cough, cold, etc. Zingiberone present in it is beneficial in rheumatoid arthritis.

15. Harad

It throws out toxic substance from the body and facilitates the working of organs properly. It provides immunity. Usually it is taken for stomach related disease but it is beneficial in other disease also.

16. Kalaunji

It is a digestive and an appetizer. It removes stomach pain and gas. It provides power to the nervous system. It regulates the menstrual cycle. It is best for sexual power and memory power.

17. Mustard Seed (Rai)

It falls in the category of mustard (Sarson). Its seed is small and black. It has a special type of pungent smell. Its main property is that it is digestive. It has the property to bring sourness. It is a pain killer.

18. Nutmeg (Jaiphal)

It is a fragrant fruit. It is hot and makes the voice melodious of a sour throat. It removes Kapha, smell in stool, worms, cough, vomiting, respiratory disorder and heart-related disease. It a is pain killer.

19. Piyalseed (Chiraunji)

It is oily, cool, sweet, a sperm enhancer, Vata, Pitta remover, thirst quencher, and power-provider for the nervous system. It is nutritious, a diuretic and beneficial for the heart. It cures burning sensations and ulcer. It removes cough. It heals the mouth sour/ulcer. It makes the skin colour fair. It is a blood purifier.

20. Saffron (Kesar)

It is hot, fragrant and a gas remover. It has vapourative (volatile) oil. Its main property is to purify the blood.

21. Salt

Natural salts in vegetables get destroyed when they are cooked. So a small quantity of salt should be used in them. But it should not be used in uncooked food such as fruits, salad, juices, etc. Use of excess salt for a long time gives birth to different diseases.

22. Turmeric

In turmeric, an element named curcumin is found which gives yellow colour to the food. It is an antibiotic, anti-inflammatory and antioxidant as well. It is Tridosha (Vata, Pitta, and Kapha) remover. It protects the liver as well as rejuvenates it. It removes constipation. It empowers the digestive system. It protects from allergy. It purifies the blood. It is very much beneficial for the skin. It is also useful in ulcer and cancer. The elements Curcumin and Turmerin present in it strengthen the immune system and protect DNA.

Those food which demands water after their consumption are harmful to humans.

Food Harmful for Health

Use of fast food like, preserved (packed) food, soft drinks, ice creams, chocolate, toffees, bread, junk food, etc., is rapidly increasing instead of natural food cooked at home. These food items are attractive and easy to use but also costlier and harmful for the body. These food items are like slow poisons which destroys our body and mind. Chemicals used in them give rise to different diseases. Some chemicals are preservatives and some are mixed for artificial fragrance and taste. Some chemicals are mixed so that stale food appears fresh. Some chemicals among them may be stored in the fat of the body for a long time which increases the possibilities of deadly disease like cancer.

To make food items attractive, different chemicals are used which increase the possibility of mouth ulcer, indigestion, throat pain, black patches on the body and asthma. It increases the possibility of liver cirrhosis.

Some Chemicals used for artificial taste

Cherry flavour – Benzaldehyde, benzoic acid, ethyl alcohol, etc.
Pineapple flavour – Ethyl butyrate.
Grapes flavour – Methyl anthranilate, amyl butyrate.
Banana flavour – ISO amyl acetate with ethyl alcohol.
Strawberry flavour – Ethyl, methyl phenyl glycidate.
Raspberry flavour – Ionone
Butter flavour – Diacetyl.
Apple flavour – Amyl valerianate with other chemicals such as ethyl alcohol, glycerine, tartaric acid, chloroform, etc.
Coffee flavour – Benzyl benzoate, ethyl acetate.
Cola flavour – Caffeine, glycerine.

These chemicals are found in soft drinks, cold drinks, drinks in closed cans and closed bottles. These give rise to ulcer, colitis and sinusitis diseases.

Use of Different Chemicals and Their Affect

Phosphoric Acid

It reduces calcium from the teeth and bones. Memory power decreases and immune system also weakens. Diseases like asthma arthritis, diabetes, etc., may appear. It is used in sugar, vegetable ghee, soft drinks and other cold drinks.

Sodium hydroxide (Caustic Soda)

It creates burning sensation in the digestive system and ulcer. It may lead to fibrotic growth. Extracts of it are found in refined oils and vegetable ghee.

Sulphur dioxide gas

It is a very poisonous gas. It is an allergenic. It weakens the immune system. It is used in sugar and refined oil formation.

Formaldehyde

It hardens the tissues. It gives burning sensation to respiratory and digestive system. It destroys kidneys. It also gives burning sensation to eyes, nose and throat. It harms the nervous system. It may lead to cancer. It is used in the formation of sugar. It is also used as a preservative. It is also found in tooth paste and shampoo.

Monosodium glutamate

It is also known by the name of Ajinomoto, Ascent, Vetsin. It damages the brain. It gives burning sensation. It gives rise to the diseases like headache, chest ache, excessive sweating, allergy, etc. It is used in fast food to make it tasty and to show the stale food as fresh.

Sodium Benzoate

It disturbs the balance of sodium, potassium and sodium phosphorus in our body. It increases the blood pressure. It is used as a preservative.

Oxalic acid

It increases acidity. It is used to increase the taste.

Caffeine

It brings genetic changes in the body. It also harms the structure of DNA and RNA and its effect can be seen in future generations. It causes nausea, sleeplessness, indigestion, stretch in muscles and mental disturbance. It stimulates the nervous system. It is used in soft drinks, chocolate, etc. It is also found in tea, coffee and tobacco.

Saccharine

It is a synthetic sweet substance which is also known as sugar free food. It is 500 times sweeter than sugar.

It is fatal for kidney and pancreas. It is cheaper than sugar so used in soft drinks, cold drinks, beverages, etc.

Soft Drinks

Different kinds of chemicals are mixed in soft drinks which are harmful to health. Soft drinks weaken teeth and bones as they absorb calcium from the body. Human teeth which does not decay if buried in soil for years, gets decayed only in 20 days if put in soft drinks. Toilets will get cleaned like with acid if soft drinks are put in them for 1 hour.

These soft drinks cause diabetes, blood pressure, insomnia, headache, stomachache, acidity, obesity, etc. They are harmful to heart and liver.

Preserved Food

A man becomes a victim of constipation, piles, sore in intestine, eye disease, blood pressure, heart disease, cancer, etc., due to the chemicals present in preserved food. They have ill effect on kidneys also.

Fast Food and Junk Food

They also have the chemicals like ajinomoto or mono sodium glutamate which slowly stores in body. So the whole body becomes toxic. It increases the possibility of cancer. It is also harmful for intestine, liver and kidney. It harms the eyes. Children suffer from asthma and continuous headache. Memory can weaken.

Persons having such food become violent and may have mental disorders. Obesity increases which results in high blood pressure, heart diseases, diabetes, etc.

Ice Cream

Instead of milk and cream, oil and water is used in formation of ice cream through western techniques. Milk is in very small quantity. To make it soft, stabilizers are mixed in it. It also has many chemicals, e.g. propyline, glycol aldinate which is a pain killer and germicide. For taste and fragrance piperonal is mixed which is a lice killer.

White Bread

It has no fiber. Lack of fiber results in constipation, diabetes, heart disease, cancer and digestive disorder. To make bread soft, tasty and to preserve it for long time chemicals are mixed. These are harmful to health.

Chocolate

It has lead which stops the growth of children. Cavity starts in the teeth even in the age of 7-8 years.

Note – There are so many other chemicals which are used in food substances for different purpose which are fatal for our body.

Hot or cold food should not be taken. Such food is harmful to health and has a bad effect on the digestive system.

Organic Food

Now-a-days different pesticides, insecticides and chemicals are used to yield high quantity crops. There is no doubt that use of these chemicals yield fast harvest and there is no harm from insects, yet entry of these chemicals in our body pose a great harm to our health.

Some crops are grown naturally without using any chemicals. Such grown crops are called organic food.

Under organic food product, all types of pulses, vegetables, flour, spices can be purchased. As organic farming process is lengthy and costly so these products are costlier than other.

Onion, ginger, garlic and coriander grown by organic way if used in right proportion can double the taste of food. If they are used in place of dry spices they increase the nutrition of the food. This is why organic food items are being used much nowadays.

It is essential to be happy while eating. It is better not to take food if feelings like anger, depression arise during food times. Food consumed during such a mental state is harmful.

Appropriate Food During Summer and Winter

Appropriate food in summer

We should take more watery food and less solid food during summer, i.e. 80% meal should be fruit and vegetables and 20% should be sprouted cereals, pulses and giri.

Best fruit and vegetables in summer season — Watermelon, melon, cucumber, papaya, mango, sapota, mulberry, pomegranate, pineapple, bael, etc.

Benefit of uncooked food in summer season —

1. protects us from heat waves
2. prevents excess perspiration and smell in sweat.
3. protects us from scorching heat
4. prevents frequent thirst
5. there is no need of air conditioner and cooler.
6. prevents the skin from sun burn.

Appropriate food in winter

In winter season watery food (fruit, vegetables and juice) should be 50% and solid food should be 50%.

Best Food and vegetables in winter season — Orange, papaya, apple, sapota, banana, carrot, tomato, cucumber, amla, cabbage, peas, etc.

Best solid food of winter season — Dates, black raisin, raisin, fig, sesame, groundnut, walnut, almond, pistachio nut, cashewnut, sprouted cereals and pulses.

Benefits of uncooked food in winter season—

1. No feeling of excess cold. Natural warmth continues in the body.
2. Prevents winter diseases (cold, cough, asthma, vata dosha, arthritis, etc.).
3. No cracks on hands, feet, skin and no dryness on skin.
4. Softness and glow of skin continues.

Food Classification

Food is divided into three categories —
(1) **Tamsik Food or Vicious Food** — The food which is partially spoiled, in which important element has got destroyed, which is cooked for a long time and preserved in such a manner that necessary life element has been destroyed is called tamas food.

E.g., meat, egg, putrid food, stale food, spicy food, too hot or cold food, fried food, packed food, tobacco, etc. It gives rise to cancer, heart related disease, ulcer, etc.

(2) **Rajsik food or Royal food** — Food which is sour, salty, very hot, spicy are royal food.

For example, junk food, sweets, namkeen, tea, coffee, soft drinks, fast food, spicy vegetable, puri, pan masala, wine, etc.

This type of food creates a strong stimulation which dominates increasing the working of uncontrolled impulse and desires which results in pain and diseases.

(3) **Satvik Diet or virtuous Diet** — Those foods which enhance long life, power, health, happiness, affection and are full of nutrition, easy to digest are satvik food.

E.g., fruits, vegetables, leafy vegetables, juices, sprouted cereals and soaked dry fruits. This food cures diseases and provides a disease free life.

Whatever we eat directly affect our body, behaviour and soul.

Types of Food

Food is life for all living beings. All are dependent on food for life, prosperity, pleasure, satisfaction, body-nutrition, power and intellectuality. If it is taken in a wrong way it may be harmful. So it becomes important to know that which food should be taken in which form, so that it becomes beneficial for the body. On the basis of softness, solid, semi-solid and liquid food, it can be divided into six categories.

(1) **Sipable** — those food which are consumed by sipping, e.g. sugar cane, orange, etc.
(2) **Drinks** — drinkable food, e.g., juices.
(3) **Lickable** — which are consumed by licking, e.g. honey, chutney.
(4) **Soft Chewable** — which can be chewed easily, e.g. pulpy fruits.
(5) **Mild chewable** — which are eaten after breaking by teeth or by cutting or by chewing, e.g. fruits, vegetables, etc.
(6) **Chewable** — it is consumed by chewing properly, e.g. groundnut, sprouted cereals, etc.

The first food is easy to digest then second, third, fourth, fifth and sixth is the heaviest to digest.

In our daily life all food should be taken in right proportion.

Six Tastes

Nature has given us six tastes which are found in different eatables. All parts of our body remains balanced if these tastes provide nutrition to them in the right proportion. By using a taste for a long time, some defects occurs in our body which results in different diseases.

	Taste	Source
1.	Sweet	Cereals, seeds, pulpy fruits, dates, honey.
2.	Sour	Sour fruits, lemon, orange, tomato, curd, butter milk.
3.	Salty	Salt, green leafy vegetables.
4.	Pungent	Chilli, spices, onion, garlic, radish, ginger, cloves, cardamom.
5.	Bitter	Spinach, turmeric, fenugreek, bitter gourd, giloe.
6.	Astringent	Cabbage, amla, alfalfa, black berry, pulses, beans/legumes.

All taste should be in right proportions in our food for being healthy. First four tastes may bear disease. Last two tastes are disease removers. During illness, for blood purification these two tastes help. Use of these two tastes in our daily diet is a must. Fenugreek seed, fenugreek water, sprouted fenugreek, amla powder, amla water can be use alternatively for these two tastes.

Seven Coloured Food

Natural coloured eatables (fruits, vegetables) has phytonutrients and pigments in large quantity. These acts as antioxidants. These prevents our DNA from getting damaged.

By enhancing S.O.D. enzymes, they increase the passion, youthfulness and life. They stop cross linking of cells which create many diseases and ageing. Persons suffering from cancer, lungs diseases, liver problems, kidney diseases, diabetes, bones diseases, eye diseases, heart diseases and other degenerative diseases can rejuvenate their life by consuming various coloured fruits and vegetables.

There are various types of phytonutrients which have different properties. If we consume foods of seven colours daily, we shall get various phytonutrients which will keep us disease free and protect various cells, tissues and organs from degenerating.

Eatables of different colours

White — Banana, pears, radish, onion, potato.
Red — Tomato, water melon, apple, strawberry, cherry, carrot, small jujube, pomegranate, beetroot.
Green — Cabbage, grapes, Chinese gooseberry, pistachio nut, peas, bottle guard, green leafy vegetables, (spinach, green coriander, mint, etc.), green bengal gram, guava, cucumber.
Blue/Violet — Falsa, black berry, brinjal, purple grape, prune.
Brown — Sapota, dates, dry dates, moth, raisin, black raisin, groundnut, almond, bengal gram, cherry, walnut, honey, alfalfa, fig, ragi.
Orange — Orange, fresh apricot, mango, rasp berry, loquat, corn.
Yellow — Papaya, pineapple, ginger, raw turmeric, lemon sweet lemon, mango, bael, jujube, melon, peach.

Malnutrition

A fast starts when you leave the food and ends when you consume the food and starvation starts when actual hunger starts and end in death.

During fasts, the body eats toxic substances present in the body and during starvation, the body eats itself.

Malnutrition is that condition when body does not get carbohydrates, proteins, fats, minerals, and vitamins in adequate proportion. It is present in a higher percentage among females.

Causes of Malnutrition

(1) Insufficient supply of food.
(2) Weak digestive system.
(3) Use of such food containing less nutrients but tastes only.
(4) Over eating.
(5) Excess cooking, frying, roasting, of food which destroy the important nutrients.

Effects of Malnutrition

(1) During malnutrition, cells weakens slowly in their working hence becomes the cause of contagious diseases like cholera, plague, T.B. and other internal diseases.
(2) Malnutrition causes body weakness which results in night blindness, beriberi, scurvy, rickets, tooth decay, osteoporosis, constipation, burning sensation in body, irritation and other diseases.
(3) It reduces the growth rate in children so possibility of low intellectual growth may increase.

Prevention from Malnutrition

(1) Use uncooked food in excess like seasonal fruits (guava, pears, papaya, etc.), vegetables (spinach, bathua, carrot, etc.), sprouted food and soaked groundnut, juice etc.
(2) Foods must be chewed properly.
(3) Avoid over eating.
(4) In case of anaemia take wheat grass juice.
(5) Use green leafy vegetables to remove iodine deficiency.
(6) Use milk of white sesame to remove calcium deficiency.
(7) Have sun bath to prevent rickets.

Artificial vitamin and minerals pills are harmful. These nutrients should be taken from the natural food item (fruits, vegetables, sprouted food, etc.). In natural food vitamins and minerals found with other micronutrient substances are much beneficial than the synthetic ones.

Keeping Fruits and Vegetables Fresh for long period

(1) Keep two or three pieces of garlic with potatoes to keep them fresh for a longer time.
(2) Bananas blacken if kept in the fridge as it is. Keep them in a glass jar and they will remain fresh for longer time.
(3) To keep radish fresh for long time, remove all its leaves except one.
(4) Keep half ripened papaya wrapped in a paper. It will ripe soon.
(5) To keep the banana fresh wrap them in wet cloth and keep in a polythene bag.
(6) Mint kept in a jar remains fresh for a longer time.
(7) Keep green coriander in an air tight jar then keep it in fridge.
(8) Keep two or three pieces of cloves among dry fruits to keep them outside the fridge.
(9) To keep lady fingers fresh, cut it from both side and keep in fridge.
(10) Lemon kept in a water jar remains fresh for longer time if water is changed daily.
(11) Hung ripened bananas remains fresh for longer time.
(12) Broken coconuts in summer season rot soon. Keep it in water and change the water regularly. It will not rotten up to 3-4 days.
(13) Keep salad leaves between two thick wet clothes.
(14) Dry fruits remain fresh for longer time in the fridge.
(15) Spinach kept in the fridge remains fresh for 5-6 days.
(16) Keep a dry sponge among the vegetables in the fridge. Squeeze it after 2-3 days; then again keep it with

vegetables. This way, vegetables remain fresh for longer time.
(17) Peeled garlic in a polythene bag kept in the fridge does not dry soon.
(18) Fresh vegetables wrapped in paper kept in fridge remain fresh for longer time.
(19) Keep cauliflower in an open polythene bag, keeping its stem upward. Make 4-5 pin holes in bag for air to pass, and then keep it in the fridge. It will not blacken soon.
(20) Keep dried vegetables in a water vessel and add lemon juice in it. Vegetables become fresh again.
(21) To be able to extract a full coconut, keep it in hot water for five minutes.

Importance of Peels of Fruits and Vegetables

(1) Use mint leaves and grow them by putting the stem in flower pots in one's own house.
(2) Wash brass utensils with lemon peels. They will shine.
(3) Wash rice in water and use this water for planting or gardening. Plants will grow faster.
(4) Dry orange peels and make its powder. Mix it with sandal powder and milk. Use it over face and neck. Skin will start glowing.
(5) Clean your utensils (like tawa and other) with a spare pulp of tamarind. They will shine.
(6) Skin remains soft if rubbed with lemon peels.
(7) Rub lemon peels on your nails and teeth and they will shine.
(8) Coriander leaves, mint leaves and other vegetables are good manures. Put them in plants.
(9) Utensils with fats can be cleaned more effectively by lemon peels.
(10) Make a powder of dried peel of lemon and orange. It will serve as a good tooth powder.
(11) Boil the water and add some pomegranate peels in it. Gargle with it. It removes bad smell from mouth.

(12) Wash copper utensils with lemon peels.
(13) Make powder of dry orange leaves. Add some coconut oil in it add some gulabjal (rose water). Face mask is ready. Use it to keep your skin soft for longer time.
(14) Keep dry peels of bitter gourd in pulses, bengal gram flour (Besan), white flour (maida), etc.; they remain preserved for longer time.
(15) Mirrors start shining after being cleaned with potato peels.
(16) Keep dry peels of lemon in the almirah. It protects clothes from worm and insects.
(17) Put peels of small cardamom in tea. It tastes better.
(18) Save peels of ripe mango; burning them keeps the mosquitoes away.
(19) Burning of banana peels in evening keeps the environment pure and good fragrance prevails everywhere.
(20) Put the peels of orange and lemon in bathing water. It gives a nice scent after bath.

Special Tips

(1) If the curd has become sour put plenty of water in it. Throw this water after 3-4 hrs. There will be no evidence of sourness.
(2) Put pieces of cauliflower in salty water. Hidden worms will come up above the water after some time.
(3) Put 3 or 4 cloves in sugar cane. It prevents ants from entering in side.
(4) Keep the butter in water at home and keep changing the water every day.
(5) Keep margosa leaves in cereals. It stays for a longer time.
(6) Wash and clean the fruits thoroughly before keeping them in the fridge as usually fruits are eaten directly after bringing them out from the fridge.
(7) Keep strawberry, mulberry, and raspberry without washing as they get putrefied if put after washing.
(8) Put crystals of salt in pulses. They remain for longer time.
(9) Pills of mercury in cereals and pulses keep them safe for longer time.
(10) If fenugreek leaves are added in wheat, it remains safe for longer time.
(11) Keep a crystals of salt in choker it is safe for a longer time.
(12) Curd formation takes longer time in winter season. Keep it on a stabilizer, curd will form quickly.

Consuming stale food is harmful. Especially students and those who are doing mental work should leave it immediately. It brings about laziness and reduces the memory power.

Importance of Style of Eating

To be healthy, eat only when you feel an actual hunger and chew it properly.

Assign two timings- morning and evening for the meals. Avoid eating at multiple times. By eating frequently in an uncontrolled way, food does not get digested properly. This undigested food is harmful.

Chewing in hurry means disregarding teeth and is hard on the intestine. Well chewed food becomes easily digestible. Unchewed food increases the load on stomach and intestine.

Digestion of starch present in food starts in mouth with the help of saliva, otherwise it increases the load of digestion for intestine. It results in a weak intestine.

When unchewed food enters the stomach then the stomach has to do the work of teeth. In the stomach, food cannot be crushed as by teeth, so stomach secrets more acid. It results in acidity and other stomach diseases.

That food which is less chewable should be kept in mouth for longer time, so that saliva mixes with it properly.

To think that overeating results in healthy body is wrong.

The stomach cannot perform in a good way when it is overloaded. Hence problems like indigestion and acidity starts. Undigested food is just as poisonous and diseases start from here.

Immunity Power

Causes of lack immunity
1. Smoking
2. Wine
3. Drugs
4. Tension
5. Inadequate sleep
6. Steroids
7. Too much use of sugar and salt
8. Lack of vitamins and minerals
9. Use of saturated and transfats oils
10. Doing more work than capacity
11. Extreme weather

Ways of enhancing immune power
1. Regular exercise, yoga, etc.
2. Long deep breathing in fresh air
3. Adequate sleep
4. Compatibility of work and rest
5. Less use of salt and sugar
6. Use of uncooked food (fruits, vegetables, sprouted cereals, soaked dry fruits, seeds, etc.)

Calories

Unit to measure the energy present in a food item is called calorie. One calorie is that amount of heat which increases the temperature of one gram of water from 14°C to 15°C. Calorie is a small unit to measure the energy present in food items, so we use kilo calorie which is equal to 1000 calorie.

We need energy to survive and to do our daily routine work. Overeating results in extra energy to store in the form of fat in our body. This gives obesity to our body.

To look slim and healthy we have to maintain a balance between energy consumed and energy absorbed by our body.

Daily need of calorie depends on height, weight, age, sex, and way or working.

700 K calorie more than our requirement increases our weight by 100 gm.

A lazy man consumes 1 K calorie per hour.

A normal man consume 3 K calorie per hour.

A very active person consumes (during running, swimming, etc.) 6 K calorie per hour.

Daily Requirement of Average Calories

Age	K. Cal. requirements per day
Children	
Up to six month	120 K. Cal. per 1 kg. weight
7-12 months	100 K. Cal. per 1 kg. weight
1-3 years	1250 K. Cal.
4-6 years	1700 K. Cal.
7-9 years	1950 K. Cal.
Boys	
10-12 years	2200 K. Cal.
13-15 years	2500 K. Cal.
16-18 years	3000 K. Cal.
Girls	
10-12 years	2000 K. Cal.
13-15 years	2200 K. Cal.
16-18 years	2200 K. Cal.
Men	
Doing Light work	2200 K. Cal.
Doing medium work	2800 K. Cal.
Doing heavy Work	3400 K. Cal.
Women	
Doing light work	1900 K. Cal.
Doing medium work	2250 K. Cal.
Doing heavy Work	2950 K. Cal.

Change is also Necessary in the Kitchen

Indian kitchen science is the most prosperous one in the world. Different kinds of food items like sweets, pickles, jams, and other dressed food are prepared in the Indian kitchen. But this is giving harm to our body. It is the misuse of money, labour and time.

This is due to our kitchen science that we are taking milk by boiling to till it become thickened (khoya) and we use it fondly. Khoya is nothing but just like the coal of milk. We use sweets made of khoya and maida interestingly which are indigestible and give rise to different diseases. The same thing goes for fried and roasted items.

We deteriorate the natural form of food to make it tastier but this is something like changing living things into non-living things. By frying, roasting and mixing spices it may become tasty but from the health point of view it will be useless and a waste.

Frying, roasting and use of excess spices should be banned in kitchen. If sweets, dressed food and spicy items are considered non-foods, it will be a boon for health.

In the modern world there are three types of kitchen—

(1) **Natural kitchen**—Nature has given cereals, fruits, vegetables, etc. If a man uses them in their natural form then he will be healthy, disease free and live a long life. Only man cooks food for his own. Other animals use food in their natural form. That is why a man falls sick frequently.

(2) **Man made kitchen**—In which food is cooked by three types—

- (a) By cooking in steam — It falls in the second category as compared to uncooked food. Mostly nutrients do not get destroyed by this way of cooking.
- (b) By boiling — This process comes in third category. Most of the nutritious elements get destroyed by this process.
- (c) By frying, roasting, using excess of salt — this falls in the fourth category. This is the most harmful process for the health.

(3) **Machine Kitchen** — Food prepared in factories in which preservatives, transfats, etc., are in plenty, are harmful for the health. They are tasty only but lack in nutrients.

When we are determined that use of natural food is necessary for our good health, then there will be a revolution in our kitchen.

The food which brings laziness and heaviness in the stomach eats you while the food which brings freshness and activeness, is eaten by you.

Effects of Non-Vegetarian Food

Man is not non-vegetarian. Structure of his teeth, salivary glands, small intestine, and other digestive organs do not resemble with that of a non-vegetarian. Nature has made him a vegetarian. An enzyme known as uricase isn't secreted in humans which is necessary to convert uric acid formed by non-vegetarian food into allentoin and carbon dioxide.

So excess uric acid is stored in a non-vegetarian's body which gives rise to arthritis, etc. A man can pass all his life without non-vegetarian food, but cannot live his whole life only on non-vegetarian food. Non-vegetarian persons have a short life whereas vegetarians have a long life. A non vegetarian is not healthy or powerful, he is weak and sick. A non-vegetarian gets tired easily whereas a vegetarian works for longer time.

Non-vegetarian food is acidic. It reduces our immunity system, which results in different diseases.

A non-vegetarian is prone to heart disease and may suffer from cancer. It increases mental problems; irritability, anger, etc., and patience power decreases. The propensity of sexual urges and agitation increases. It is believed to increase aggression.

Survey shows that among criminals, number of non-vegetarians are more than vegetarians. Non-vegetarian food give rise to tamsic propensity leading to incidents of mental differences, domestic squabbles, fights, etc. Egg is also a non-vegetarian food. It is believed to be full of cholesterol in a very dangerous form which is responsible for heart diseases.

In eggs, a substance known as Avidin is found which destroys a part of B-complex known biotin. It reduces mental and physical growth. Although Westerners are generally non-vegetarians, they are now converting to vegetarianism.

Adulteration in Food Stuff and Detection

Pure and fresh food is necessary for a healthy body and healthy mind. Different foods are being adulterated directly or indirectly.

Affect of adulteration, is seen in the body gradually which results in various diseases. Today everyone is on the verge of falling sick by eating this adulterated food. Due to this, different bad results like nervous breakdown, epilepsy, weak vision, asthma, allergy, skin diseases, etc., are coming.

Different sweets, ice creams, toffees, pills, spices, pulses or other food items are coloured with some artificial colours. Synthetic colours are also used in some food items to make them attractive. All these coloured items are poisonous and can damage DNA of cells which may result in cancer. These coloured food items may bring about genetic change. Chromosome and genes are also affected by them. Liver, kidney, skin and lungs are badly affected by these artificial synthetic colours. So avoid artificially coloured food items.

In mixed item (spices, etc.) cheaper constituents are increased and costly parts are decreased which make them less effective. So it is better to make such mixes at home.

Calcium carbide is used to ripen fruits and vegetables. So fruits and vegetables must be used after proper washing. Cereals and pulses must be used after wash.

We can be safe from adulterated food by the following tips of detection.

S.No.	Food	Items	Adulteration Detection
1.	Milk	Water	Put one drop of milk on a smooth surface. If it flows without leaving behind any spot then water is mixed. If it flows slowly leaving behind a white line then it is pure.
		Starch, urea or other chemicals	Put some drop of iodine solution in the milk. If colour changes to blue then it is adulterated.
		Sodium Bicarbonate (Meetha soda)	Take 3 ml of milk. Add 10 drops of rosalic acid. If colour changes to pink it shows the mixing of sodium bi-carbonate.
2.	Khoya and its other items. Chhaina or Cheese	Starch or chemicals	Take a little of these product. Boil it in water. Then allow cooling. Add some drops of iodine in it. If the color changes to blue then it is adulterated.
3.	Ghee, Butter	Vegetables,	Take one spoon of ghee or margarine or butter. Add same quantity of concentrated hydrochloric acid. Add a little sugar in it. Mix it well for one minute. Keep it for five minutes. If a dirty cream color appears at bottom layer then vegetable oil, or margarine is added.

Adulteration in Food Stuff and Detection

S.No. Food	Items	Adulteration Detection
6. Jaggery	Sodium Bicarbonate	Take a piece of 5 gm in a test tube. Add 3 ml of hydrochloric acid in it. Appearance of froth is evidence of adulteration.
7. Honey	Sugar solution	Soak a ball of cotton with honey. Burn it. If honey is pure cotton will burn easily. If it is adulterated it will not burn. Even if still it burns a cracking sound appears. Add one drop of honey in water. If it dissolves, honey is adulterated other wise it is pure. A fly comes out of some drops of pure honey if put on it. Dog does not lick the pure honey.
8. Sweets, Ice-cream other drinks	Saccharin	Saccharin mixed food and tastes sweet in the beginning but later it leave bitter taste on the tongue.
9. Sella Rice (Parboiled rice)	Metanil Yellow	Rub some grains of rice with hands. It loses its (A non-yellow color. Put some permitted drop of dilute coal-tar hydrochloric acid and colour) some water in it. Appearance of pink color is the evidence of metallic yellow.

S.No. Food	Items	Adulteration Detection
10. Turmeric	Metanil	Take small spoon yellow turmeric in a test tube. Add some drops of concentrated hydro-chloric acid in it. Instant appearance of yellow color shows that turmeric is pure. If it persists it shows mixing of metanil yellow.
11. Gram Powder (Besan)	Khesari Powder	Add 50 ml of dilute hydrochloric acid in 10 gm of besan. Boil it for 10 minutes. If pink color appears then besan is adulterated with khesari powder.
	Metanil	Take half spoon of yellow sample in a test tube. Add 3 ml. wine in it. Shake it well. Add 10 drops of hydrochloric acid in this solution. If it turns pink, then it is adulterated.
12. Kesar (Saffron)	Dried tendrils of maize cob	Pure kesar leaves its colour gradually till it gets dissolved completely. But adulterated kesar leaves the colour immediately.
13. Vinegar	Mineral Acid	Dip metanil yellow indicator paper in vinegar. If it turns pink it indicates the adulteration.

Adulteration in Food Stuff and Detection

S.No.	Food	Items	Adulteration Detection
14.	Coffee	Chicory	Take a glass of water. Sprinkle some coffee powder on it. Pure coffee powder floats over water. But chicory sinks in few seconds. It also leaves some colour on sinking.
		Crushed seed of tamarind or dates	Sprinkle coffee powder over a bloating paper. Put 1% sodium carbonate solution. Adulterated sample leaves red spots on blotting paper.
15.	Tea leaves	Exhausted tea or gram dal husk with Color	Put the tea leaves over a soaked blotting paper appears on paper colour if it is adulterated tea.
16.	Green Vegetables	Malachite Green	Rub the vegetable with a cotton soaked in liquid paraffin. If white cotton turns green it is adulterated.
17.	Red Gram Dal (Arhar Dal)	Khesari Dal	Structure of Khesari Dal is like a Pentagon. It can be separated by looking carefully.
18.	Powder of	Powder of	Put half spoon of the coriander wood sample in half water or cumin bowl. Pure sample sinks but wood powder floats on the water surface.

S.No. Food	Items	Adulteration Detection
19. Black Pepper	Seeds of	Float the sample in papaya alcohol. Pure pepper Light black sinks whereas papaya pepper seed or light pepper floats on the surface. Papaya seed are odorless and small in size. It can be separated by looking smelling and examining.
20. Red chilly	Rodamine-B	Rub the sample with (dry) color cotton soaked in liquid paraffin. If it turns red then the sample is adulterated. If the sample leaves red color on putting over a wet blotting paper then it is adulterated.
21. Red Chilly powder	Colored wooden	Put the powder in water. If color dissolves in it powder then it is adulterated.
22. Asafoetida	Soapstone or other earthy matter.	Put the asafoetida in water then shake it well. Adulterated asafetida sinks down.
	Starch	Put some drops of iodine. If asafoedita turns blue then it is adulterated. If it gives smell on putting in fire then the sample is pure otherwise not. Pure asafoetida changes the color of water to milky.

S.No. Food	Items	Adulteration Detection
23. Cloves	Volatile oil	Evaporated cloves are extracted small in size and get (Exhausted shrunk. The pungent cloves) taste in pure cloves is not in evaporated cloves.
24. Cinnamon	Peels of	Rub it with hands if guava stem adulterated no colour appears.
25. Common salt	Crushed white stone or chalk powder, etc.	Dissolve one teaspoon of salt in a glass of water. If adulterated it will turn milky and other non-dissolving items settle at bottom.
26. Silver leaves	Aluminum	On burning, pure silver leaves foil leaves behind a shining ball of same size whereas aluminum foil leaves behind an ash of dark brown color.

Poisonous Atmosphere

There is a danger for human beings from poisonous chemicals. Different diseases like headache, irritation, chronic physical and mental disorder and indigestion are spreading rapidly. Heart disease and cancer are also increasing.

Carbon Monoxide

This is the most dangerous part in polluted air which gives maximum harm to health. It blocks haemoglobin in red blood cells 250 times faster than oxygen. Hence there is no adequate supply of oxygen to our body. It results in different diseases of lungs ulcer, headache, shortness of breath, suffocation, anaemia, heart and cancer diseases. It comes out from smoking tobacco, gas, wooden or kerosene stove and from improper chimneys.

Lead

It is found in increasing quantity in air, water and food. It is a very fatal element. It can harm even if it is in a very small quantity. It comes from lead gasoline mainly, but also comes from lead ceramic glaze and other commercial products.

Lead is a stored poison. It is basically incurable. It causes lack of appetite, fatigue, and weak nervous system. It also harms kidney liver and heart. It may cause wounds in intestine, paralysis, blindness, menstrual disorder, schizophrenia and mental problems. It may also cause anaemia, impotency, sterility and abortion. It is also be harmful to pregnant women.

It stops growth in children and causes nervous and mental imbalances.

Calcium protects the digestive system from its poison. It stops and removes the poison of lead.

Mercury

This is an abandoned poison in our present environment. It has polluted the earth, water and eatables. It is a stored poison. It damages the brain and nervous system. It also damages kidney and liver. It may cause blindness or paralysis.

D.D.T.

These days D.D.T. is present everywhere. Although the American government has restricted the use of it, yet it is being used in developing countries on a large scale. Even if its use is stopped immediately, yet it would remain in the environment as it has been used on a very large scale earlier. It is stored in the fat fibers in our body. Reducing weight fast may be fatal as then D.D.T. may get separated from the fat and may harm our body system badly. Hence weight should be reduced slowly.

Cadamium

It is useful in its natural form in a very small quantity, but is fatal for air pollution. It is found in smoke coming out from engines. It is also found in gasoline and lubricants oils. Usually it is found in phosphate fertilizers and pollute the earth. From there it enters in vegetables and cereals.

This poison also enters in our body when we use cadamium galvanized utensil. This poisonous cadmium is used to give an attractive shine to utensils.

For health it is more dangerous than lead.

It may cause high blood pressure, and heart disease. It may also lead to anaemia, kidney diseases, lungs disease and suffocation. Stancium-90

This poison arises during nuclear testing. Scientists say that if stancium-90 is already present in the human bone, it remains in the body for whole life.

Radio Active Iodine

It is very dangerous. It may be more poisonous than stancium-90. Mostly it is found in milk, hence it may harm those who drink milk.

In our body system, radio-active substances get stored rapidly. Mainly it is stored in the thyroid gland. When its quantity increases then it causes throat cancer.

Oxone and Nitrogen dioxide

These are air polluting fumes which cause harm to our health. It causes irregularities in the respiratory system especially suffocation.

X-Rays

Doctors, dentists and orthopedicians use X-Ray. But we cannot neglect its harmful effect. Overexposure to X-Ray leads to leukaemia and other cancers; X-ray exposure to a pregnant woman's abdomen may lead to leukaemia in the mother and child also.

Poisonous Affects of Medicine

All chemical medicines are poisonous in little or large quantities and their effects are harmful. At least 10% of the sick patients are because of medicines. Even over use of aspirin affects millions of persons and kills hundreds of them.

Many medicine reacts with vitamins in our system. These bring irregularities in our metabolism and body functions. Medicines destroy minerals and vitamins and prevent them from assimilation. Many medicines damage the liver and kidney badly. Even impotency, sterility and cancer may appear.

Chemical medicine should be taken only in emergency under the supervision of a skilled doctor.

Nitrates and Nitrites

Many food items, flesh, etc., are preserved by these chemicals. They are also used for colouring fresh flesh. Nitrate is also used in fertilizers. This way these pollute the earth and water also.

These are highly poisonous. These may lead to different diseases of the liver, stomach, oesophagus, urinary bladder, kidney and heart.

Nitrates and Nitrites prevents kerotine from converting them in vitamin A. They also destroy stored Vitamin A in the body system.

General Sources of Prevention Against a Poisonous Environment

1. Go outside the polluted city and be in the fresh air for some time and keep a fast on juices.
2. Take wheat grass juice.
3. Use fruits and vegetables after washing well and clean.
4. Use curd or butter milk.
5. Use food rich in Vitamin A, B, C, D, E and calcium.

In the present era, only uncooked food (fruits, vegetables, sprouted, etc.) is the cheapest, universal and easiest way to protect from a poisonous atmosphere.

Enhancing Beauty through Fruits, Vegetables and Juices

Beauty is that which comes from the inside. Beauty is not which needs a polish from the outside. A natural glow, freshness and attraction appears on the face by using green vegetables, salad, fruits and juice regularly.

As a result of good health, the skin remains beautiful and fresh and glowing forever. Artificial make-up is for a small time and it harms the skin also.

Artificial beauty enhancers in market are costly and harmful. Use of homemade tips for enhancing beauty is the best as they are not only cheap but do not harm the body. They do not give a temporary glow to the skin but is everlasting.

General food items like fruits, vegetables, and juice have been used to enhance beauty since ancient times.

(1) Make the paste of an apple and apply it on the face for 10-15 minutes. It makes the skin soft. It tightens the skin and reduces oil of the face.

(2) Apply ripened banana on the skin and throat for 15-20 minutes. Rub it with tissue paper. Wash it with fresh water. It gives nutrients, freshness and softness to the skin.

(3) Extract juice from cabbage leaves. Add little honey to it. Apply on the skin and throat. After 15 minutes, sponge it with wet cotton. It removes the spots on the face. It is very useful to cure acne. It stops dryness, wrinkles, and reduces blackish colour of skin. It stops skin infections.

(4) Peel a pear. Apply its pulp on the face. Wash after some time, it removes skin dryness.

(5) Grind the mint leaves and apply them on acne face. It gives relief.
(6) Grind an unripe papaya. Apply the paste on the face. Wash it after 15 minutes. It gives relief in acne and hyper pigmentation.
(7) Add few drops of lemon juice in one spoonful of tomato juice. Apply it on face. Wash after 15 minutes. It removes spot and patches from face.
(8) Use grapes juice every day on face. Wash after 10 minutes. It makes skin glow, shiny and gives nutrition to the skin.
(9) To get rid of sun burn in summer season, use coconut water on the skin. It will bring glow and fair colour to the skin.
(10) Grind the cucumber and keep it in the fridge to cool. Use it in this way twice a week on the face. Wash the face with cold water after 15 minutes. It brings freshness and gives relief from scorching sun.
(11) Add turmeric in tomato juice or beet juice. Drinking it improves the skin color.
(12) To remove wrinkles from the face, use ground sprouted wheat with milk on the face.
(13) Use of carrot juice daily removes skin dryness.
(14) In winter season use of tomato juice daily removes skin diseases and dryness.
(15) Apply pulp of pumpkin on the neck. It removes its blackish color.
(16) Apply melon pulp on the skin, it makes the skin clear and removes the smell of sweat.
(17) Massage of falsa juice on lips makes lips more beautiful and attractive.
(18) Rubbing teeth with peels of sweet lime removes their filth.
(19) Sun burned skin get relief when juice of carrot or cucumber mixed with rose water is applied on it.

(20) To clean up make up, wash face with cotton soaked in milk.
(21) Dry the peels of lemon, sweet lime and orange. Grind them. Mix them with a little gram flour (besan). Add gulabjal in that. Apply on the face. Remove on drying by rubbing with hands and wash with lukewarm water. It helps in removing hair from the face.
(22) Cut the pieces of cucumber. Put those on the eyes. It gives cool feeling to the eyes. Bags under eyes also disappear.
(23) Add Multani Mitti (yellow mud) in cucumber juice. Apply on face and neck. It gives relief to oily skin and also cleanse the skin.
(24) Applying the paste of cucumber, milk, lemon and honey brings is good for the face.
(25) Drinking juice of carrot and tomato increases blood quantity in the body and is good for skin.
(26) Add the juice of one lemon and one spoon of honey in tomato pulp. Apply it on the face. Rub for some time. It makes the skin charming.
(27) Use of coconut water with cucumber juice on the skin having spots and patches, is very beneficial. It makes the skin better.
(28) If small pores appear on the face use tomato juice mixed with half lemon juice. Rub it slowly. On drying repeat the process. Wash after some time. Do it for 15 days.
(29) Mix one lemon juice in a bucket of water for bath. It keeps the skin fresh.
(30) For dark lips—mix two spoon of lemon juice in one spoon of pure honey. Apply it on the lips in morning and at night while sleeping.
(31) Use almond oil on dry lips at night. It makes them softer. Never scratch the dry layer on lips with nail or teeth.
(32) To enhance the beauty of nails, dip them in milk for some time.

Enhancing Beauty through Fruits, Vegetables and Juices

(33) If the nails are brittle and weak, apply lemon juice with cotton on them and rub the nails with peels of lemon. Wash the hands after some time.

(34) Having beet salad daily, enhances the beauty of unhealthy and yellowish nails.

(35) Rubbing milk on the body removes dryness of the skin and skin begins to glow.

(36) Use raw milk on the lips with cotton. It removes blackish color of the lips.

(37) Dissolve rice flour in milk. Use it on the face. It removes the wrinkles from the skin and makes the skin softer.

(38) Grind Harsingar flowers, white flour (Maida) and milk together. Use this paste on the skin. Skin becomes soft and fragrant.

(39) Mix Multani Mitti (yellow mud) in milk. Apply it on the face and body. It gives coolness and prevents prickly heat in summer season

(40) Grind the raw coconut in milk. Use this paste on face, neck, hands and legs. It makes skin fair and smooth.

(41) Grind basil leaves with milk, and apply it on the face. It removes pigmentation.

(42) Rub nutmeg with milk. Use this on the face. It removes pigmentation and acne of the face.

(43) Make a paste of milk cream and honey. Use this paste below eyes. It removes the bags under eyes. Use of it on lips prevents them from drying and cracking and makes them beautiful.

(44) Massage of almond oil on the skin not only keeps it soft but also removes wrinkles.

(45) Grind piyal seeds with milk. Use it on the face. The skin improves.

(46) Use the paste of basil leaves on face, half an hour before bath regularly. It makes the skin charming as basil has a natural bleaching agent.

(47) Any type of spot on face can be removed by using nutmeg rubbed with coconut water regularly and

washing in the morning with cold water. Use it for six weeks. It gives expected benefit.

(48) Use curd on the face once a day and wash it after 20 minutes. It removes black heads from the face.

(49) Eat four pieces of garlic on an empty stomach. It tightens the droopy breasts.

(50) Mix olive oil with double quantity of buffalo milk. Apply it on the breasts half an hour before the bath. It makes the breasts sturdy.

(51) Use coriander juice on lips to make them softer.

(52) To remove dark circle around the eyes apply coconut oil. Dark circle will disappear in few days.

(53) Clean the hair with Multani mitti (yellow mud) mixed with salt and oil. It helps to remove dandruff from the hair.

(54) Use lemon juice at the root of hair to strengthen them. After that wash them with Multani mitti (yellow mud). It makes hair stronger and dense too.

(55) Multani mitti (yellow mud) enhances the beauty of hair. Mix Multani mitti (yellow mud) with curd, then wash the hair with it.

(56) Mix gram flour in juice of carrot. Apply it on the face. It removes pigmentation and wrinkles.

(57) Mix Multani mitti (yellow mud) in orange juice. Apply it on the face. It removes skin dryness.

(58) Dissolve the pulp of pear in raw milk. Rub this paste with cotton on the face. Then wash the face with lukewarm water. Skin glows like a fresh flower.

(59) Mix lemon juice in the curd. Apply this on skin. The dull skin becomes alive.

(60) Rubbing a piece of ripened papaya on the face removes dirt, blackishness and wrinkles from the face.

(61) Cut the potato in circular pieces. Put them on the eyes. It reduces the swelling of eyes.

(62) Mix lemon juice in coconut water. Apply it on hair. It removes dandruff.

Enhancing Beauty through Fruits, Vegetables and Juices

(63) Apply mint leaves juice on face to remove spots and for clean skin.

(64) Rub the peel of lemon on finger. It removes their blackness.

(65) Mix half spoon of lemon juice with half spoon of honey. Apply it on the face for 10 minutes. Wash the face with cold water. Do it twice a week. Face will glow.

(66) Apply the juice of orange on the face for 10 minutes, Then wash. It clears the skin colour.

(67) Clean your face with raw milk twice a day. It improves the skin colour. Skin becomes soft and smooth.

(68) Grind the basil leaves in lemon juice. Apply this paste on face. It removes all the spot, patches and pigmentation from the face.

(69) Cucumber has some elements which makes the hair dense. Apply cucumber juice in the roots of hairs and then wash with water. It nourishes the hair. Regular use of it makes the hair dense and long.

(70) Add 4-5 drops of lemon juice in a table spoon of cucumber juice. Add a little turmeric powder in it. Apply this paste on the face and neck. Let it dry. After half an hour wash the neck and rub with thick towel. It is good for the skin.

(71) Never use soap or shampoo to wash the hair. Wash the hair with lemon juice water (1/2 lemon juice in 1 glass of water). It clears the dandruff. Hair becomes dense and long.

(72) Grind the petals of red rose. Add a little glycerin to make it paste. Apply this on lips at night. It changes the color of lips from blackish to red. Already red color lips become redder.

(73) Apply lemon juice with glycerin in same proportion at the dry elbow. It becomes softer in few days.

(74) If the nails are hard and painful on cutting, dip them in water for some time. You can cut easily.

(75) Apply mustard oil in the navel to prevent the lips from cracking.
(76) If the eyes have become deep and blackish colour appears below the eyes, then keep almond oil and honey mixed in same proportion. Massage around the eyes with this before going to sleep. It is instant relief providing. Instead of almond oil with honey, olive oil alone is also beneficial.
(77) Massage from nose to eye with dry palm. This fills the dip on cheeks. In the beginning do it for 10-15 times, later increase the practice.
(78) Grind the petals of rose in milk. Apply it on face. It is good for the skin.
(79) Add fenugreek powder in myrtle (Mehandi). It will give dark color.
(80) Rub the nails with alum. They will be strong and shiny.
(81) Grind the green coriander leaves. Mix lemon juice in it. Unwanted moles disappear.
(82) Rub the peel of lemon on elbow. It removes their roughness and blackness.
(83) Grind almond nut in raw milk. Apply this on face. It is good for the skin.
(84) Drinking tomato juice, mint juice and lemon juice together removes acne (pimples) from the face. Skin colour improves.
(85) Mix barley flour, sesame oil, and turmeric together. Make a paste. Use it on the face. The face becomes soft and shiny.
(86) Soak the rose petals, black raisin, almond and nutmeg in milk for the whole night. Make a paste of it by grinding in the morning. Apply it on the face. Regular use of it removes the pigmentation and moles from the face.
(87) Mix one spoon of tomato juice, half spoon of lemon juice, a little turmeric powder and a little gram flour to make a paste of it. Apply it below the eyes on black circles for 10 minutes. Massage gently and then wash

with simple water. Use it once a day regularly for few days. This is most effective way to remove black circles around the eyes. For fast relief, drink tomato juice.

(88) Mix 100 gm of curd with one spoon of orange juice and one spoon of, lemon juice. Apply this on the face for 15-20 minutes. Wash the face in lukewarm water. The face becomes shiny.

(89) In a bowl of curd, add half spoon lemon juice, little Multani Mitti and apply this paste on the face as a face pack for 15-20 minutes. This is best remedy for dry skin.

(90) Make a paste of two spoon lemon juice, one spoon almond oil, two spoon wheat flour, and one spoon curd. Apply it on hands, legs, face and neck. After 5 minutes, remove by rubbing in reverse direction. Get rid of unwanted hair on the skin. The skin will glow.

(91) Squeeze one lemon in half a cucumber. Add a little turmeric and a spoon of honey in it. Make a paste by grinding. Apply it on the face, neck, hands and legs. Wash after 10 minutes. Continue for a week. It removes pigmentation, blackness below the eyes and improves colour of skin.

(92) Take 16 spoon of gram flour, half spoon of turmeric powder and a little raw milk. Make a paste. Add 8-10 drops of mustard oil or olive oil. Stir it till it becomes a paste. Apply this on face, neck, hands, legs and all parts of the body. Let it dry for some time. After this, remove the paste by applying pressure through hands (by rubbing). Paste comes out like small wicks along with the dirt. Now after some time wash it with lukewarm water or take a bath. Dry the body with a towel. The skin becomes clear, as smooth as silk, as soft as butter and face will be shiny. Applying this paste on the face removes pigmentation, spot, wrinkles and blackish of the face. It removes the unwanted hairs from the face.

> There is no cosmetic for beauty like happiness.

Balanced Diet

The main constituents of diet are—(1) Protein, (2) Carbohydrate, (3) Fat, (4) Vitamins, (5) Natural salts, (6) Fibre, (7) Water

Each constituent is as necessary as the other as they are dependent on each other for their performance. So it becomes necessary to add these constituents in our diet in a proper way. Generally nature provides all necessary elements for our body in each food items, but some constituents are in less quantity in a food item and other are in plenty. So it becomes necessary to know which food item contains which element and in what proportions. Accordingly we should create our diet.

Protein

This is necessary for development of body and for daily compensation.

Deficiency of Protein

Its deficiency causes problems like fatigue, weakness, retarded development, nervous weakness, etc. In pregnancy, the mother's and foetus's tissues become weak. The body may collapse before time due to lack of protein.

Excess of Protein

As lack of protein creates problems, similarly excess of protein is also harmful. Problems created due to lack of proteins can be solved by giving extra protein. But problems created by excess of protein will require complete cleansing of the body.

Excess of protein affects liver and kidney. Uric acid stores in joints leading to gout and rheumatoid. It contaminates the blood. Arteries and veins are blocked with waste deposits leading to pressure on blood circulatory system. Heart becomes weak. Due to high blood pressure sometimes blood vessels may burst and result in paralysis. Apart from these many minor ailments occur due to excess of protein.

Sources of Protein

Milk, dry fruit, dual seed grains, peas, green leaves, etc., and soya bean are the richest in protein.

According to work done, generally an adult needs 50-60 gm of protein every day. Approximately the proportion should be one gram of protein per kilo of weight.

Children, athletes, pregnant and breast feeding women need more protein.

Amino Acid—It is one of the constituents of protein. There are about 80 types of amino acid, out of which 20 are essential for human metabolism or for growth and development. Some of them are automatically formed in the liver and others, are called essential amino acid.

These are—(1) Arginine, (2) Cystine, (3) Histidine, (4) Isolucine, (5) Leucine, (6) Lysine, (7) Methionine, (8) Phenylalanine, (9) Threonine, (10) Tryptophan, (11) Tyrosine, (12) Valine.

These are provided by different food items like cereals, pulses, leafy vegetables etc.

Amino Acid Charts

Amino Acid	Function	Sources	Deficiency	Recommended Daily Allowances (RDA)
(1) Arginine	For development, for immune system for detoxification, for the metabolism of muscles, for making insulin, effects the pancreas.	Milk, groundnut, cashewnut, watermelon seeds, walnut, green vegetables, root vegetables, coconut, sprouted wheat, soya bean	Impotency, sterility, high blood pressure, heart disease.	Not established
(2) Cystine	It contains sulphur. Necessary for nail, hair and skin. Help in detoxification. It acts as antioxidant. Prevent arteries from hardening.	Milk, Banana, Grapes, fig, dates, seed of sunflower, green leafy vegetables, ragi etc.	General Weakness	Not established

Amino Acid	Function	Sources	Deficiency	Recommended Daily Allowances (RDA)
(3) Histidine	For the development and maintenance of tissues. To convert glucose into glycogen in liver. In forming RBC and WBC	Fruits (banana grapes etc.) milk, green vegetables, root vegetables.	Joints pain, Rheumatic arthritis.	Not established
(4) Isolucine	To regulate the work of thymus, spleen and pituitary glands. Help in formation of haemoglobin.	Pulses, soya bean, milk, cashew nuts, and cereals.	Hypoglycemia	12 mg. adult 28 mg. Children 80 mg. infants
(5) Leucine	Regulate the metabolism of protein in the body	Milk, whole cereals, pulses, soya bean and leafy vegetables.	—	16mg Adult 42 mg. child 128 mg infants

Amino Acid	Function	Sources	Deficiency	Recommended Daily Allowances (RDA)
(6) Lysine	Stops the growth of viruses and throws them out. Formation of muscles. Enhance concentration and collegen	Leafy vegetables, pulses, beans, milk, ripe fruits, soya bean.	Low appetite, loss in weight, headache, nausea, malnutrition, acid fomentation in blood, irritation	12 mg adult 44 mg child 97 mg Infants
(7) Methionine	Protect liver, reduce cholesterol, assimilate fat, necessary for balancing the body weight, helper in detoxification, work as an anti-oxidant	Whole cereals, milk, curd, leafy vegetales, grapes, garlic, onion, seeds, soya bean.	Swelling in Kidney	10 mg Adult 22 mg; child 45 mg; Infants
(8) Phenyla-lanine	Regulate appetite, helps in balance the body weight, help in functioning of kidney and urinary bladder, activate the mood.	Milk, curd, pulses, whole cereals, leafy vegetables, groundnut, almond, pistachio nuts, peas, soyabean.	Cataract, reddish eyes, depression	16 mg Adult 22 mg Child 132 mg. Infants

Amino Acid	Function	Sources	Deficiency	Recommended Daily Allowances (RDA)
(9) Threonine	For the development and function of mind, help to protect stiffness, reduce fats from liver, immunity enhancer.	Leafy vegetables, whole cereals, groundnut, soyabean, nut, pulses, fig, apple, un-polished rice.	Irritability in children.	8 mg Adult 28 mg Child 63 mg Infants
(10) Triptophan	Essential for blood clotting and formation of digestive juice, stops premature ageing, reduce tension. Help in sound sleep.	Vegetables, seeds, nuts, soyabean, groundnut,	Pellagra, increased sensitivity to light	3 mg Adult 4 mg Child 19 mg Infants
(11) Tyrosine	Keeps mood charming, reduce tension, reduce fat, help in the function of adrenal thyroid and pituitary glands.	Milk, wheat, banana, grapes, dates, fig, seeds, of sunflower, leafy vegetables, apple, soyabean raagi.	Depression	—

Amino Acid	Function	Sources	Deficiency	Recommended Daily Allowances (RDA)
(12) Valine	For proper functioning of nervous system, prevents digestive and nervous disorders, important for body growth.	Milk, leafy vegetables, cereals, pulses, cashew nuts, nuts, groundnuts, soyabean.	Sensitive to touch and sound.	14 mg Adult 25 mg Child 89 mg Infants

(2) Carbohydrates

It gives us strength and heat.

Deficiency of carbohydrates

Deficiency of carbohydrates cause laziness, inactiveness and lethargy.

Excess of carbohydrates.

Excess of carbohydrates increases obesity. It gets accumulated in the breathing pipe, stomach, intestine, heart and uterus in the form of toxins and gives rise to various diseases.

It has two parts – (1) starch (2) sugar

Starch

The food which is sticky is rich in starch. Every starch converts into sugar after complete digestion and stored in liver and muscles as glycogen. Scientist has divided them in to three categories.

(1) Easily digestible (Alkaline) – It is found in banana, potato, sweet potato, papaya, pear, sapota, orange, apple, pineapple and guava.

(2) Easily digestible (Acidic) – It is found in rice, barley, maize and other tuber root.

(3) Late digestible (Acidic) – it is found in all types of single seed grains (wheat, jowar and bajra or millet.) Removing bran from these, change them fully in acid.

Sugar

It is of five types –

(1) Milk Sugar – This is required much during pregnancy. It is found maximum in human milk.

(2) Grape Sugar – It is found in grapes of high quality, honey and in other fruits. Scientists have called it predigested food, as the digestive system has to do no work to digest them. That is why honey or raisin water is given as a source of instant energy.

(3) **Fruit Sugar** — Usually it is found in all sweet fruits. In the plant juice, it is found as glucose. When the fruits ripen, starch converts into sugar. So we should eat always ripe fruits, otherwise we will get acid instead of alkaline from the fruit. For a diabetic patient, fruit sugar is more harmless than the other one (white sugar). Its digestion occurs in small intestine.

(4) **Malt Sugar** — It is found in daily eaten starchy cereals like — wheat, barley, rice, maize, etc. In spite of the sugar they are rich in salt, calcium, iron, etc., and vitamins too. Its digestion starts in the mouth with saliva and completed in the small intestine.

(5) **Cane Sugar** — It is the sugar made from sugar cane. It has the ability to provide heat. It is highly acidic. It is of low level and harmful. The more we try to whiten the cane sugar, the more it loses its nutrients like calcium, iron, other natural salts and vitamin.

To digest sugar and to compensate the lost nutrients, the digestive system takes calcium and iron from our body. As a result, the body starts lacking in these items. Although this affects the bones of our body, yet its direct effect is in decay of teeth. Eating excess sugar produces oxalic acid which has no use in our body. When adequate calcium is not found to digest sugar then it creates havoc in the body.

After having learnt this much, the question rises, what is the substitute of sugar. The answer is sugarcane, jaggery, dates, raisin, banana, fig and mango, sweet fruits as available in season.

Generally an adult should take 200-500 gm of carbohydrates according to his physical work.

(3) Fats

Like carbohydrates, fats also provide heat. It is the best food to provide energy. It is useful to make the skin smooth and to strengthen the bone. Without sugar, fat is not oxidized properly and continue to burn which causes tiredness in the body. To digest fats, the liver, pancreas and intestine should be in sound condition. For this, deep breathing in open air is necessary. Excess of fat gives birth to different diseases, and its deficiency is compensated by the body from other food.

To activate fat in our food, iodine is necessary, otherwise the disorder in the thyroid results in goitre. It is divided into two parts
   (1) Vegetable generated — It is found in every oil, sesame, mustard, olive, sunflower, groundnut, linseed, etc., dry fruits (coconut, almond, walnut, cashew nut, pistachio nut, piyalseed and pine fruit etc.)
   (2) Animal generated — Milk and its product. First kind of fat in goat milk, second in cow milk, and third type in buffalo milk.

Types of fats

Fat is triglycerides. It is made of one molecule of glycerol and three molecule of fatty acid. it is of two types
(1) Saturated, (2) Unsaturated.
   (1) **Saturated fats** — it solidifies at normal temperature. It is mostly found in vegetable generated fat. It is not beneficial for the body as it increases bad cholesterol and decreases good cholesterol in body.
   (2) **Unsaturated fats** — it is in liquid form at normal temperature. It regulates the blood cholesterol. It is generally found in vegetable oils. It is also of two type —
   (a) Mono Unsaturated (b) Poly Unsaturated
      (a) **Mono Unsaturated** — The body generates them itself, as per requirement. So it is not an essential fatty acid. It falls in the category of Omega-9.
      (b) **Poly Saturated** — These are essential fatty acid and need to be extracted from the food. It falls in the category of Omega-3, and Omega-6.

Fats Chart

	Saturated	Mono unsaturated	Poly unsaturated
Butter	54.0%	28.0%	2.5%
Coconut oil	85.2%	7.8%	2.0%
Corn oil	12.7%	29.6%	57.4%
Cotton seed oil	25.9%	22.9%	50.9%
Ghee	65.0%	29.0%	Nil
Groundnut oil	20.9%	49.3%	29.8%
Hempseed oil	10.0%	15%	75%
Mustard oil	10.7%	56.0%	32.6%
Olive oil	14.8%	74.5%	10.0%
Palm oil	46.3%	43.7%	10.0%
Rice bran oil	22.1%	41.0%	35.7%
Canola oil	5.3%	64.3%	24.8%
Safflower oil	10.7%	16.7%	73.5%
Sesame oil	13.7%	41.3%	44.5%
Soya bean oil	13.1%	28.9%	57.2%
Sunflower oil	9.1%	25.1%	66.2%
Wheat germ oil	18.8%	15.9%	60.7%

Essential Fatty Acids (EFA)

These are important for the health but cannot be generated by the body. So they are called essential fatty acids. These are poly unsaturated fatty acids.

Functions of Essential Fatty Acids

(1) These activate exocrine and endocrine glands.
(2) These are helpful in forming Haemoglobin.
(3) Provides lubrication to the joints.
(4) Functions to carry the cholesterol.

Balanced Diet

(5) For regular pulsation of heart, they help to generate electricity.
(6) Helps the immune system.
(7) Prevents growth of allergy.
(8) They contribute in every activity of the body.

Important fatty acids are of two types—
(1) Omega-3, (2) Omega-6

Omega - 3 — Deficiency of omega-3 causes —
(1) Retarded growth in infants, children and pregnant women.
(2) Blood pressure increases.
(3) Possibilities of blood clots increase.
(4) Triglycerides and cholesterol. (LDL) increases.
(5) Heart pulsations become irregular.
(6) Concentration and memorizing power decreases.
(7) Menstrual problems increase.
(8) Problems of vision.
(9) Immunity power decreases.
(10) Feeling of shivering in hands and legs.

Sources of Omega-3—dark green vegetables, linseed, cloves, walnut, pumpkin, sprouted wheat, soya bean, unpolished rice, nuts, etc.

(3) Omega-6—Deficiency of omega-6 causes—
(1) Arthritis.
(2) Behavioural changes
(3) Skin and hair gets dry
(4) Dryness and itching in eyes.
(5) Skin eruptions like eczema starts.
(6) Hair fall starts.
(7) Retarded growth.
(8) Heart pulsations becomes irregular
(9) Wounds take time to heal
(10) Pre menstrual syndrome starts.
(11) May get infectious diseases.

Sources of Omega-6 – Walnut, pumpkin, grapes, sunflower seed, sprouted wheat, maize, sesame, groundnut, almond, soya bean, unpolished rice.

Chart of Essential Fatty Acid

Food	Omega-3	Omega-6
Almond oil	0%	17%
Cashewnut oil	0%	6%
Corn oil	0%	59%
Flax seed oil/Linseed oil	58%	–
Flax seed/Linseed	15.3%	–
Grape seed oil	0%	71%
Groundnut oil	0%	30%
Hempseed oil	20%	60%
Mustard oil/Rapeseed oil	7%	30%
Olive oil	0%	8%
Pumpkin seeds oil	15%	50%
Rice Bran oil	1%	35%
Safflower oil	0%	75%
Fish Salmon oil	30%	0%
Sesame oil	0%	45%
Soya bean oil	7%	51%
Sunflower oil	0%	65%
Walnut oil	11.5%	58%
Wheat Germ oil	5%	50%

Trans Fats

Trans fats are very harmful to the body. They give birth to many diseases. They increase bad cholesterol and reduce good cholesterol. They increase obesity and diabetes. They are mainly manmade.

When vegetable oils are converted into refined oils by chemical process, they get converted into trans fats. Oils also get converted into trans fats when they are boiled or fried. 4% trans fats are also found in animal milk.

Balanced Diet

So oil should not be used in cooking or frying. Requirement of oil in the body can be fulfilled by uncooked food, by just eating a piece of coconut, some groundnut, walnut or some sesame.

(4) Vitamin

Vitamins are those organic substances which are essential for many activities of the body. They can be obtained from the food.

Vitamins in the food get destroyed by boiling excessively or by cooking in a wrong way.

Vitamins are classified in two groups.
  (1) Water soluble — As the body cannot store them, so their daily supply to the body is essential like vitamin B complex, vitamin C, vitamin U, etc.
  (2) Fat soluble - The body can store them. They are vitamins A, O, E, F, P, etc.

Our body has the capacity to generate some vitamins. There are some useful bacteria in our intestine which secretes vitamin for the body. They are vitamins B, E and K. Antibiotic medicines destroy these useful bacteria hence there may be deficiency of these vitamins in the body after the use of antibiotics.

All vitamins get destroyed in little or more proportion due to heat, by coming in contact with air or due to storage of food. Vitamin C is destroyed very quickly.

Vitamin A can bear a little heat but during open cooking it gets destroyed immediately.

Vitamin Chart

Vitamin	Function	Sources	Deficiency	Recommended Daily Allowance (RDA)
1	2	3	4	5
Vitamin-A (Retinol) (Carotene)	For healthy skin and eye sight, for immune system.	Milk, butter, green leafy vegetables, red or yellow fruits (Mango, papaya, banana, alfalfa, tomato, carrot, etc.)	Night blindness, low appetite, eye, nose and skin diseases, possibilities of bacterial infection.	1-1.5 mg.
Vitamin-B Complex Vitamin-B-1 (Thiamine)	This is essential to convert carbohydrate into energy, essential for heart muscle and nervous system.	Milk, whole cereals and pulses, green leafy vegetables, nuts.	Beriberi, heart and mental diseases.	1-1.4 mg.

1	2	3	4	5
Vitamin B-2 Riboflavin	Necessary to all cells for energy and maintenance, eye sight, nervous system	Milk, soyabean, sprouted wheat, green leafy vegetables, papaya, banana, kiwi, alfalfa.	Mouth ulcer, less appetite, weakness in neuron system, skin disease, cornea, opaqueness	1.2-1.7 mg.
Vitamin B-3 Niacin (Nicotinic acid or Nicotinamide)	Essential for digestive system and nervous system, to convert food into energy.	Whole cereals, pulses, nuts, tomato, banana, water melon, pea, carrot, alfalfa generated by intestinal bacteria.	Ulcer of mouth and tongue, diarrhoea, mental disorder, skin diseases.	13-19 mg.
Vitamin B-5 (Pantothenic acid)	For converting food into energy, help in making adrenal hormone and good cholesterol.	Milk, whole cereals, pulses, groundnut, green leafy vegetables, orange, banana.	Tiredness, muscles weakness, disorder in the function of adrenal glands and nerve cells.	4-7 mg.

Vitamin	Function	Sources	Deficiency	Recommended Daily Allowance (RDA)
Vitamin-B-6 (Pyridoxine)	Help in the formation of RBC, help in proper functioning of nervous system and formation of antibodies, metabolism of protein.	Milk, sprouted wheat, green leafy vegetables, pulses, soyabean, groundnut, maize, alfalfa, banana.	Diseases of eye, nose, ear, mouth and skin. Problems related to blood vessels and nerve tissues, nausea.	0.3-2 mg.
Biotin	Necessary for skin and blood circulatory system.	Nuts, fruits, vegetables, generated by the intestinal bacteria.	Depression, pain in muscles, tiredness, nausea.	0.06 mg.
Vitamin B-9 (Folic acid) (Falate)	For the formation of nucleic acid (DNA and RNA) required for RBC. For the development of embryo, essential for pregnant lady.	Green leafy vegetables, fruits, whole cereals, nuts, generated by intestinal bacteria.	Anaemia, sterility, underweight of infants.	0.4 mg.

1	2	3	4	5
Vitamin B-12 Cyanocobalamin	Necessary for the formation of RBC, bone marrow and DNA. For nervous system.	Milk, sprouted wheat, alfalfa, soyabean, peas.	Anaemia, low appetite, tiredness, (lack of it is rare).	0.003 mg.
Vitamin-C (Ascorbic acid)	For healthy teeth, bone and gums. Enhance the blood vein. Faster healing of wounds. Prevents internal bleeding. Keeps skin healthy. Gives resistance power. It acts as antioxidant.	Citrus fruits, tomato, cabbage, gauva, amla, green leafy vegetables, papaya, mango, sprouted cereals.	Teeth diseases, pyorrhoea, scurvy, blood pressure and bleeding, ageing before time.	45-60 mg.

Vitamin	Function	Sources	Deficiency	Recommended Daily Allowance (RDA)
Vitamin-D (Calciferol) (Cholecalciferol)	For healthy teeth and bone. For the assimilation of calcium and phosphorus.	Milk, sprouted seeds, vegetables with wide leaves, dry fruits ripen in sun (almond, chilgoza, walnut, etc.), sunflowers seed, formation by skin in the sun light.	Osteoporosis, muscles weakness, nervous system weakness, ricket in children, muscular cramps.	5-10 mg.
Vitamin-E (Tocopherol)	Necessary for normal reproductory function, normal development, necessary for blood veins and blood circulation.	Milk, whole cereals, sprouted wheat, peas, groundnuts, green leafy vegetables, tomato, dry fruits, soya bean, cabbage.	Infertility, impotency, premature birth of baby, low blood pressure, liver disorder.	8-10 mg.

1	2	3	4	5
Vitamin-F	For skin, nervous system, endocrine glands, prostate gland.	Seeds, uncooked Alsi and its unrefined oil.	Hormonal imbalance	Not established.
Vitamin-K	For clotting	Green leafy vegetables, cabbage, groundnut, soya bean, tomato, green grass (Dooba), fresh fruits and vegetables, walnut, spinach.	Bleeding	1.5-5 mg.
Vitamin-P	For the healthy blood vessels and to maintain normal blood pressure.	Fresh fruits and vegetables, walnut, spinach.	Weekened blood vessels results in bleeding, tiredness.	Not established.
Vitamin-U	Provides protection to intestinal membrane.	Fresh vegetables, cabbage.	Membrane of digestive system weaken.	Not established.

Natural Minerals

These are essential for cleansing, construction and development of the body. These are also essential for the assimilation of food. There is no part in the body which can function without natural minerals. No gland, no part of digestive system and no digestive juice in the body can perform properly the functions of blood circulation and nerves impulses, without the help of natural minerals..

Out of different elements, essential elements for a normal body are as follows:

1. Calcium 1000 gm
2. Phosphorus 780 gm
3. Potassium 140 gm
4. Sulphur 140 gm
5. Sodium 100 gm
6. Chlorine 95 gm
7. Copper 72 gm
8. Magnesium 19 gm
9. Iodine 13 gm
10. Manganese 12 gm
11. Iron 4.2 gm
12. Fluorine 2-6 gm
13. Zinc 2.3 gm
14. Chromium 2.0 gm
15. Cobalt 1.5 gm

Minerals Chart

Minerals	Function	Sources	Deficiency	Recommended Daily Allowance (RDA)
1	2	3	4	5
1. Boron	It regulates the use of calcium, phosphorus and magnesium. Control cell growth, prevent abnormalities in growth.	Fruits, vegetables, especially apples, pears and carrot.	Tumors, cysts	2 mg.
2. Calcium	Essential for bones and teeth. Essential for activity of enzymes in the body. For nervous system. For heart and all muscles, for embryo development, for electrically active cells or tissues in body. For blood clotting.	Milk, sesame, green leafy vegetables, cabb-age, tunip, beet, orange, water chestnut (singhada), masoor pulse, almond, fig, bran of cereals, water melon, dry fruits, bajra, raagi.	Bones become brittle, teeth decay, rickets, bleeding, and disturbance in heart pulsation, nervous weakness, muscles stiffness.	800-1200 mg.

Minerals	Function	Sources	Deficiency	Recommended Daily Allowance (RDA)
3. Chlorine	It cleans the body, blood purifier, important for secretion of digestive acid. Protects stiffness of joints.	Green leafy vegetables, grains, pulses, fruits, vegetables.	Indigestion, de-arrangement of fluid level in the body, hair fall, weight loss.	300-900 mg.
4. Chromium	Essential for the metabolism of carbohydrates, fats. To carry the protein where required.	Nuts, leafy vegetables.	Lack of protein and energy.	0.05-0.2 mg.
5. Cobalt	In the production of haemoglobin. A part of vitamin B-12.	Green leafy vegetables, guava, carrot, beet.	Deficiency of it in the body is rare	Not established

1	2	3	4	5
6. Copper	It works with iron for the formation of haemoglobin. Important for the use of vitamin C.	Whole cereals, iron containing food, water chestnut, se-same, walnut, cashew nut, groundnut.	Anaemia, respiratory disorder, general weakness, limited development and growth.	1.5-3 mg.
7. Fluorine	For the healthy teeth.	Bengal gram, green leafy vegetables, cereals.	Tooth decay	0.5-0.8 mg.
8. Iodine	It keeps thyroid gland healthy. It increases mental power. It prevents from goiter and obesity. It helps in oxidation of protein and fats.	Water grown crops (Lotus seed, makhana, water chestnut etc.), pine apple, green vegetables, tomato spinach.	Enlarged thyroid gland, Goitre occurs.	0.1-0.15 mg.

Minerals	Function	Sources	Deficiency	Recommended Daily Allowance (RDA)
9. Iron	It helps in the formation of haemoglobin, for immunity, prevents fatigue.	Green leafy vegetables, whole cereals, pulses, apple, dates, dry fruits, guava, banana, brinjal, apricot, raisin, grapes, carrot, coriander, etc.	Anaemia, lack of immunity and RBC, lack of haemoglobin, jaundice.	25-30 mg.
10. Magnesium	For cells, for electrical activities of muscles and veins.	Milk, green leafy vegetables, beans, water chestnut, cereals, alfalfa, walnut, groundnut.	Indigestion, tiredness, irritation, weak nervous system, weak mental power, Hearts strokes.	300-350 mg.

1	2	3	4	5
11. Manganese	It makes the nervous system strong. For the metabolism of protein, carbohydrates and fats.	Whole cereals, nuts, beat, cabbage, guava.	Indigestion, less development, abnormal grwoth of bones.	3 mg.
12. Molybadenum	Essential for metabolism, help in the formation of haemoglobin, for the assimilation of iron.	Milk, whole cereals, beans, green leafy vegetables, nuts.	Weakness, anaemia.	0.5 mg.
13. Phosphorus	Send power to cells, makes the teeth and bones healthy with calcium. Strengthen the nervous system. Essential for the development of body, metabolism, heart and liver.	Milk, whole cereals, green leafy vegetables, beans, water chest nut, dry fruits, turmeric, groundnut.	Weak teeth and bones, weight loss, rickets and weakness.	800-1000 mg.

Minerals	Function	Sources	Deficiency	Recommended Daily Allowance (RDA)
14. Potassium	For muscles. It brings flexibility in muscles and nerves. Balance the acidity in the body. Essential for brain and RBC. Strengthen the nervous system, dissolve out toxic substances from the body.	Milk, green leafy vegetables, orange, sunflower seeds, alfalfa, watermelon, white pumpkin, cucumber, cabbage, tomato, green gourd, groundnut.	Slow development, constipation, gas trouble, nervous disorder, insomnia, laziness.	1700-5500 mg.
15. Selenium	It acts as natural anti-oxidant. Keeps the tissues young, keeps away ageing.	Garlic, whole cereals (as sprouted wheat), vegetables.	Cancer, heart disease, swelling type disease, early ageing.	0.04-0.07 gm.

1	2	3	4	5
16. Silicon	For nerves and their function, for the strong bones, hairs, nails and teeth. For healing wounds.	Alfalfa, apple, sunflower seeds, almond, groundnut, grapes, green vegetables, fruits, amla.	Soft brittle nails, wrinkles on skin, excessive hair fall and greying, osteoporosis.	Not established.
17. Sodium	Balance in body fluids, essential for muscles and nervous system, essential for gastric acid.	Leafy vegetables, fruits, vegetables, pulses, beans, alfalfa.	Nausea, weakness in muscles, muscular cramps, low blood pressure, nerves disorder.	1000-3000 mg.
18. Sulphur	Blood purifier, helps in formation of bile in liver. Essential for skin, nail and hairs. For the metabolism of carbohydrates.	Green leafy vegetables, beats, cauliflower, garlic, onion, radish, alfalfa, red gram dal, water melon, tomato, fig.	Hairs and nails disorder.	300 mg.

Minerals	Function	Sources	Deficiency	Recommended Daily Allowance (RDA)
19. Vanadium	For the metabolism of sugar and cholesterol. Hence prevents heart strokes.	Cereals, vegetables, nuts, oil seeds, fruits (apple, plum etc.)	Not established.	0.0014 mg.
20. Zink	For healthy hair and skin, for healing wounds, for immune system, for carrying vitamin A to retina. For conceiving, for healthy prostate.	Cereals, nuts, oil seeds, fruits and vegetables.	Late healing of wounds, taste disorder, retardation in growth and delayed genital maturation.	10-15 mg.

Fibres

It acts as a broom in the digestive system. Cleaning of intestines is impossible without it. So its presence is necessary in our diet; lack of it causes constipation, which is the root cause of all diseases.

Sources – It is found in each type of fruits, vegetables, cereals, and flora. It mainly remains in upper parts of the food, so we should eat wheat with bran, pulses with peels. It is in plenty in isabghol bran, fig, bael and raisin.

Water

70% of our body weight (except fats) is water. Our body needs 1-7 litres of water every day. The requirements depend upon our nature of work, humidity, temperature and other conditions. On an average, a man needs 8-10 glass of water every day. Approximately 20% of water, we get from food. Other 80% is gotten from drinking juice and water.

Water comes out from the body in the form of sweat, urine, stools, and breath.

Water used for drinking and bathing should always be at the same temperature of body. Cold water damages the digestive system. During meals, we should not drink water.

Nowadays Instead of water, tea, coffee, sugar beverages and synthetic drinks are served. These are harmful to our body.

If you want to drink something else instead of water, drink fruits or vegetable juice, coconut water and other such organic juices.

Antioxidants

Antioxidants are those nutrients in our food which protect us from free radicals, and stop their formation.

Free radicals are produced during simple activities of the body. They are also generated due to tension, smoking, and consumption of alcohol, scorching sun, pollution, oily and fried food. They damage cells and tissues of our body and also harm the immune system. It results in different fatal diseases like heart diseases, ageing before time, diabetes, cataract, cancer, arthritis, brain contraction, etc. To protect this, anti oxidants are needed.

Their functions were discovered first by naturopaths, and scientific endorsement was given later in modern labs. Vitamins A, C, E and salenium and some phytochemicals also act as antioxidants. Some bodies also make enzymes work as anti oxidants.

Some antioxidants get ruined by cooking food for a long time or storing for a long time.

Sources of Antioxidants

Pomegranate, grapes, orange, pineapple, Chinese gooseberry, black plum, cherry, strawberry, raspberry, black raisin, peach, guava, pear, mango, green leafy vegetables, lemon, ginger, beetroot, cabbage, celery leaves, tomato, apricot, dates, pistachio nuts, almond, cashew, fig, soybean, turmeric, wheat grass, walnut, groundnut, sunflower seeds alfalfa, bajra, barley, oat, maize, cloves, cinnamon, whole cereals.

ORAC (Oxygen Radical Absorpancy Capacity) is the measurement for antioxidants present in any food item. A normal man needs at least 3000 ORAC per day.

Value of Antioxidants in Different Foods

Food	ORAC Per 100 gm
Raisin	2830
Black berry	2036
Cabbage	1770
Straw berry	1540
Spinach	1260
Raspberry	1220
Plum	949
Alfalfa	930
Broccoli	890
Beet root	840
Orange	750
Grapes	739
Cherry	670
Kiwi (Chinese goose berry)	602
Grape fruit	483
Onion	450
Corn	400
Brinjal (Egg Plant)	390

Different kind of fruits, salad, sprouted food, nuts, etc, fulfils the daily requirements of the anti oxidants. Instead of getting it from the supplement it is better to get from food.

Phytonutrients

They are active nutrients which are obtained from plants. They have many wonderful preventive and curative properties. They are also called phyto chemicals. They are found more in coloured fruits and vegetables. Their number is in thousands and their activities are also different.

Main functions of Phytonutrients

Antioxidant function – Many phytonutrients act as antioxidants, which protects the damage done by free radicals and prevents cancer.
Hormonal function – They prevent menopausal syndromes and osteoporosis.
Enzymes activation – They activate the enzymes.
Interference with DNA – Interfering with DNA, they stop the growth of cancer cells.
Anti bacterial effect – they kill bacteria.
Physical action – Some phytonutrients get attached to the walls of cells and protect us from microbes.

Some important Phytonutrients

Carotenoids – It prevents heart diseases, strokes, blindness and some types of cancer, reduces ageing process and complications of diabetes. It improves the working of lungs. It is found in dark red, green, yellow, and orange coloured fruits and vegetables.

There are different phyto chemicals in this group but the four main are following:
(A) *Beta Carotene* – It reduces the risk of ageing and cancer, it reduces the complications of diabetes, and improves

the function of lungs. It is found in green, yellow and orange coloured fruits and vegetables (mango, apricot, papaya, carrot, pumpkin, Chinese gooseberry (kiwi), spinach, cabbage, etc.).

(B) *Lutein* – This is essential for proper vision as we age. It reduces the risk of cataract and some type of cancers. It is found in spinach, kiwi, broccoli, mango, orange and plum.

(C) *Lycopene* – It reduces the risk of prostate cancer and heart diseases. It is found in red-coloured vegetables and fruits (tomato, watermelon, etc.).

(D) *Zeaxanthin* – It prevents visual impairment which starts after 50 years of age. It prevents certain types of cancer. It is found in maize, spinach, orange, pumpkin, cabbage.

Flavonoids – They are also called biflavonoids which act as antioxidants. They prevent cancer, ageing and heart disease. They are found in orange, kiwi, grapes, berries, broccoli, onion, etc.

There are many phyto chemicals in this group but the five main are as follows –

(A) *Resveratrol* – It reduces the risk of heart disease, cancer, blood clotting and strokes. It is found in grapes, groundnut, nuts, and seeds,

(B) *Anthocyanins* – It prevents signs of ageing (imbalances, short term memory, etc.) It also prevents urinary tract infection. It is found in black berry, cherry, strawberry, kiwi, plum, etc.

(C) *Quercetins* – It reduces the swelling associated with allergies, prevents the growth of head and neck cancer and it also protects the lungs from harmful effects of pollutants. It is found in apple, cherry, grapes, onion, cabbage, broccoli, garlic, etc.

(D) *Hesperidin* – It prevents heart diseases. It is found in fruits and their juices like orange and its juice, grapes and its juice,

(E) *Tangeritin* – It prevents cancers of head and neck. It is found in citrus fruits.

Phenolic Compounds – It reduces the risk of heart disease and some types of cancer. It enhances the immune system. It reduces the nervous weakness caused by ageing. It is found in berries, plum, grapes, kiwis, raisin, apple, tomato, etc.

The main phyto chemical of this group is –

Ellagic acid – It reduces cholesterol and prevents some types of cancer. It is found in grapes, kiwi, guava, black berry, strawberry, raisin, walnut, etc.

Isothiocyanates – It acts as antioxidants and prevents cancer. It is found in Broccoli and in other vegetables.

The following phyto chemical is important in this group.

Sulphoraphane – It reduces the risk of colon cancer. It is found in broccoli, cauliflower, cabbage, turnip, etc.

Monoterpenese – It prevents the formation of tumors and also prevents heart diseases. Useful in treating gall stones. It is found in soya bean.

The main phyto chemical in this group is –

Limonene – It protects lungs and prevents certain types of cancer. It is found in orange, grapes, lemon, sweet lemon, etc.

Indoles – It reduces the risk of certain types of cancer including breast cancer. It is found in cabbage, broccoli, cauliflower, turnip, etc. The main phyto chemical of this group is allicin.

Allium Compound – It reduces cholesterol, blood pressure. It reduces the risk of certain types of cancer. It is found in garlic, onion, green leafy vegetables.

Genistein – It reduces the growth of tumor. It is found in soya bean, soya bean milk and curd.

Polyphenols – It restores a failing immune system. It is found in sprouted wheat.

Isoflavones – It prevents osteoporosis, arteriosclerosis and heart disease. It is found in soya bean.

Saponins—It prevents the growth of cancer cell by interfering with DNA. It is found in beans.

Pronthocyanidius—It reduces the infection of urinary tract. It is found in cranberry.

Whenever you go outside your city, use amla powder. It prevents you from the complications arising from the changed weather and water of the new place.

***   ***   ***

Twist the tongue towards palate. Keep it for as long as you can. It will continue the formation of Somras and keep you healthy.

Enzymes

Enzyme is a type of catalyst. It is produced in cells. It acts as a catalyst in even a very small quantity. It encourages the chemical reaction in the body. Every reaction in the body depends upon enzymes. For every reaction in the body, one or more unique enzymes are required. In this way every enzyme has a definite work.

Every living body or vegetable cells are capable of producing enzymes.

Enzymes are of more than a thousand types. In their deficiency, life is impossible. They help in digesting the food. They break the food into their basic constituents, so that, they can be absorbed easily in the intestine. They build cells, glands and nerves from the digested food. These are the main contributors to storing glycogen in the liver. These also help in expulsion of carbon dioxide from lungs.

Some fixed type of enzymes help in storing phosphorus in bones. Some joins iron with RBC and some help in clotting of blood. There are also some type of enzymes which attack on the toxic substance and other unwanted things in the body. They change them into urea and uric acid and throw them out of the body.

Some enzymes can convert protein into sugar or fats whereas some others can convert fat into other useful substance. In reality enzymes have different functions in the body.

Enzymes have all the natural nutrients. Enzymes get destroyed on heating, still we take cooked food. That is why we do not get enzyme from the cooked food and do not live a long life.

Our body can secrete enzymes according to our requirements, but for that the concerned organ has to work hard. During young age this is easily done, but in older age, the organ gets weakened, so enzymes are not secreted according to our requirement and hence we fall sick.

If uncooked food can give all necessary enzymes easily to the body, then why should we give unnecessary burden to our body? Why do we not leave the work of reconstruction to enzymes present in uncooked food? Nature has this provision.

It has been proved scientifically that, for better performance, the body cannot do without enzymes. In inadequate supply of enzymes, the body starts degenerating. Many dieticians believe that early ageing is due to lack of enzymes.

In the older age, the body cannot produce enzymes by itself, so there is no other way than to get it from uncooked food. It does not mean that children or youth do not require uncooked food. Use of uncooked food prevent extra burden on enzyme secreting organs and they work for a long life.

Enzymes are necessary for the body and good health. They are destroyed on heat. Hence sufficient uncooked food (fruits, vegetables and juices) should be consumed.

Lecithin

It is a fatty food substance and enriched in phospholipids which serves as a saturated material for every cell in the body. It is an essential constituent of the human brain and nervous system. Lecithin is also an important component of the endocrine glands and muscles of the heart and kidneys. Nervous, mental or glandular over activity can consume lecithin faster. This may render a person irritable and exhausted. So it is necessary to add lecithin in diet.

Benefits – It is very important to the heart. It breaks the cholesterol into small parts and does not allow them to be stored in blood vessels. It is also generated in the liver, from there it goes to the small intestine with bile. It is absorbed there and comes into the blood. It helps in transportation of fats. It increases formation of bile acid from cholesterol. This reduces the cholesterol from the blood. So it is clear that cholesterol will give trouble only when there is lack of lecithin in the blood.

Lecithin in adequate quantity can regenerate those organs which need it. It reduces the process of ageing.

It is important for the medication of skin disease like acne, eczema, psoriasis. It restores sexual power. Its use is also valuable in minimising pre-menstrual and menopausal problems. It prevents the stone formation in gallbladder and dissolves it.

Deficiency – in a normal brain 28% lecithin is found and in a mentally-affected one, it is only 10-14%. So deficiency of lecithin results in mental illness.

In its deficiency, the working of endocrine glands reduces. Its deficiency can also cause infertility and impotency. Early ageing starts. Its deficiency is fulfilled by bone marrow and nervous system which results in nervous disorder.

Sources – It is found in pure vegetable oil (not in refined oil), in uncooked food. It gets destroyed on heating. It is found in plenty in soya bean, sesame, groundnut, cabbage and sprouted wheat, cucumber seeds, bottle gourd and linseeds are also good sources.

Lecithin produced in a factory should not be used.

Fruits or vegetable which look like a body organ is good	
Almond	*for eyes*
Pineapple	*for throat*
Tamarind	*for appendix*
Walnut	*for brain*
Bottle gourd	*for stomach*
Cucumber (Kakri, Tori)	*for small intestine*
Cucumber (Khira)	*for large intestine*
Bitter gourd	*for pancreas*
Amla	*for gall bladder*
Apple	*for heart*

Minerals, Vitamins, Fibre and Energy Found in Different Kinds of Food Items (in per 100 grams)

Food Items	Protein gm	Carbohydrate gm	Fat gm	Minerals gm	Calcium mg.	Phosphorus mg.	Iron mg.	Vitamin-A mg.	Vitamin-B-1 mg.	Vitamin-B-2 mg.	Vitamin-B-4 mg.	Vitamin-C mg.	Fibre gm	Energy K.Cal
	1	2	3	4	5	6	7	8	9	10	11	12	13	14
Vegetables														
Amaranth Tender	4.0	6.1	0.5	2.7	397	83	3.49	5.520	0.03	0.30	1.2	99	1.0	45
Ash Gourd	0.4	1.9	0.1	0.3	30	20	0.8	0	0.06	0.01	0.4	1	0.8	10
Banana Stem	0.5	9.7	0-.1	0.6	10	10	1.1	0	0.02	0.01	0.2	7	0.8	42
Beans	7.4	29.8	1.0	1.6	50	160	2.6	0.034	0.34	0.19	0	27	1.9	158
Beet Root	1.7	8.8	0.1	0.8	18.3	55	1.19	0	0.04	0.09	0.4	10	0.9	43
Bitter Gourd	2.1	10.6	1.0	1.4	23	38	2.0	0.126	0.07	0.06	0.4	96	1.7	60
Bottle Gourd	0.2	2.5	0.1	0.5	20	10	0.46	0	0.03	0.01	0.2	0	0.6	12
Brinjal	1.4	4.0	0.3	0.3	18	47	0.38	0.074	0.04	0.11	0.9	12	1.3	24
Broad Beans	4.5	7.2	0.1	0.8	50	64	1.4	0.009	0.08	—	0.8	12	2.0	48

Minerals, Vitamins, Fibre and Energy Found in Different Kinds...

	1	2	3	4	5	6	7	8	9	10	11	12	13	14
Carrot	0.9	10.6	0.2	1.1	80	530	1.03	1.890	0.04	0.02	0.6	3	1.2	48
Cauliflower	2.6	4.0	0.4	1.0	33	57	1.23	0.030	0.04	0.10	1.0	56	1.2	30
Cluster Beans	3.2	10.8	0.4	1.4	130	57	1.08	0.198	0.09	0.03	0.6	49	3.2	16
Colocasia	3.0	21.1	0.1	1.7	40	140	0.42	0.024	0.09	0.03	0.4	0	1.0	97
Cucumber	0.4	2.5	0.1	0.3	10	25	0.60	0	0.03	0	0.2	7	0.4	13
Drum Stick	2.5	3.7	0.1	2.0	30	110	0.18	0.110	0.05	0.07	0.2	120	4.8	26
French Beans	1.7	4.5	0.1	0.5	50	28	0.61	0.132	0.08	0.06	0.3	24	1.8	26
Jack Fruit	2.6	9.4	0.3	0.9	30	40	1.7	0	0.05	0.04	0.2	14	2.8	51
Lady Finger	1.9	6.4	0.2	0.7	66	56	0.35	0.052	0.07	0.10	0.6	13	1.2	35
Lotus Stem	4.1	51.4	1.3	8.7	405	128	60.6	0	0.82	1.21	1.9	3	25.0	234
Mango Green	0.7	10.1	0.1	0.4	10	19	0.33	0.090	0.04	0.01	0.2	3	1.2	44
Mushroom	4.6	4.3	0.8	1.4	6	110	1.5	0	0.14	0.16	2.4	12	0.4	43
Nisorha	4.7	9.3	0.5	2.6	1740	116	–	–	–	–	–	–	3.3	61
Onion	1.2	11.1	0.1	0.4	46.9	50	0.60	0	0.08	0.01	0.4	11	0.6	50
Papaya Green	0.7	5.7	0.2	0.5	28	40	0.9	0	0.01	0.01	0.1	12	0.9	27

Food Items	Protein gm	Carbohydrate gm	Fat gm	Minerals gm	Calcium mg.	Phosphorus mg.	Iron mg.	Vitamin-A mg.	Vitamin-B-1 mg.	Vitamin-B-2 mg.	Vitamin-B-4 mg.	Vitamin-C mg.	Fibre gm	Energy K.Cal
	1	2	3	4	5	6	7	8	9	10	11	12	13	14
Potato	1.6	22.6	0.1	0.6	10	40	0.48	0.024	0.10	0.01	1.2	17	0.4	97
Peas	7.2	15.9	0.1	0.8	20	139	1.5	0.083	0.25	0.01	0.8	9	4.0	93
Pumpkin	1.4	4.6	0.1	0.6	10	30	0.44	0.050	0.06	0.04	0.5	2	0.7	25
Pear Gourd	2.0	2.2	0.3	0.5	30	40	1.7	0.153	0.05	0.06	0.5	29	3.0	20
Radish	0.7	3.4	0.1	0.6	35	22	0.4	0.003	0.06	0.02	0.5	15	0.8	17
Raw Banana	1.4	14.0	0.2	0.5	10	29	6.27	0.030	0.05	0.02	0.3	24	0.7	64
Ridge Gourd	0.5	3.4	0.1	0.3	18	26	0.39	0.033	—	0.01	0.2	5	0.5	17
Snake Gourd	0.5	3.3	0.3	0.5	26	20	1.51	0.096	0.04	0.06	0.3	0	0.8	18
Sweet Potato	1.2	28.2	0.3	1.0	46	50	0.21	0.006	0.08	0.04	0.7	24	0.8	120
Sword Beans	2.7	7.8	0.2	0.6	60	40	2.0	0.024	0.08	0.08	0.5	12	1.5	44
Tinda	1.4	3.4	0.2	0.5	25	24	0.9	0.013	0.04	0.08	0.3	18	1.0	21
Tomato	0.9	3.6	0.2	0.5	48	20	0.64	0.351	0.12	0.06	0.4	27	0.8	20

Minerals, Vitamins, Fibre and Energy Found in Different Kinds...

	1	2	3	4	5	6	7	8	9	10	11	12	13	14
Tomato Green	1.9	3.6	0.1	0.6	20	36	1.8	0.192	0.07	0.01	0.4	31	0.7	23
Turnip	0.5	6.2	0.2	0.6	30	40	0.4	0.000	0.04	0.04	0.5	43	0.9	29
White Pumpkin	0.5	3.5	0.1	0.3	10	30	0.6	–	0.02	0	0.4	18	0.8	17
Yam	1.2	18.4	0.1	0.8	50	34	0.6	0.260	0.06	0.07	0.7	0	0.8	79

Cereals

	1	2	3	4	5	6	7	8	9	10	11	12	13	14
Barley	11.5	69.6	1.3	1.2	26	215	1.67	0.010	0.47	0.20	5.4	0	3.9	336
Indian Corn (Millet)	11.6	67.5	5.0	2.3	42	296	8.0	0.132	0.33	0.25	2.3	0	1.2	361
Jowar	10.4	72.6	1.9	1.6	25	222	4.1	0.047	0.37	0.13	3.1	0	1.6	349
Maize	11.1	66.2	3.6	1.5	10	348	2.3	0.090	0.42	0.10	1.8	0	2.7	342
Ragi	7.3	72.0	1.3	2.7	344	283	3.9	0.042	0.42	0.19	1.1	0	3.6	328
Rice Bran	13.5	48.4	16.2	6.6	67	1410	35.0	–	2.70	0.48	29.8	0	4.3	393
Rice Polished	6.8	78.2	0.5	0.6	10	160	0.7	0.000	0.06	0.06	1.9	0	0.2	345
Rice Unpolished	7.5	76.7	1.0	0.9	10	190	3.2	0.002	0.21	0.21	3.9	0	0.6	346
Wheat	11.8	71.2	1.5	1.5	41	306	5.3	0.064	0.45	0.17	5.5	0	1.2	346

Food Items	Protein gm 1	Carbohydrate gm 2	Fat gm 3	Minerals gm 4	Calcium mg. 5	Phosphorus mg. 6	Iron mg. 7	Vitamin-A mg. 8	Vitamin-B-1 mg. 9	Vitamin-B-2 mg. 10	Vitamin-B-4 mg. 11	Vitamin-C mg. 12	Fibre gm 13	Energy K.Cal 14
Pulses														
Bengal Gram	17.1	60.9	5.3	3.0	202	312	4.6	0.189	0.30	0.15	2.9	3	3.9	360
Black Gram	24.0	59.6	1.4	3.2	154	385	3.8	0.038	0.42	0.20	2.0	0	0.9	347
Green Gram	24.0	56.7	1.3	3.5	124	326	4.4	0.094	0.47	0.27	2.1	0	4.1	334
Horse Gram	22.0	57.2	0.5	3.2	287	311	6.77	0.071	0.42	0.20	1.5	1	5.3	321
Kidney Beans	22.9	60.6	1.3	3.2	260	410	5.1	—	—	—	—	—	4.8	346
Lentil Whole	25.1	59.0	0.7	2.1	69	293	7.58	0.270	0.45	0.20	2.6	0	0.7	343
Lobia (Cow Pea)	24.1	54.5	1.0	3.2	77	414	8.6	0.012	0.51	0.20	1.3	0	3.8	323
Moth	23.6	56.5	1.1	3.5	202	230	9.5	0.009	0.45	0.09	1.5	2	4.5	330
Red Gram Dal	22.3	57.6	1.7	3.5	73	304	2.7	0.132	0.45	0.19	2.9	0	1.5	335
Soya Beans	43.2	20.9	19.5	4.6	240	690	10.4	0.426	0.73	0.39	3.2	—	3.7	432

Fruits

	1	2	3	4	5	6	7	8	9	10	11	12	13	14
Amla	0.5	13.7	0.1	0.5	50	20	1.2	0.009	0.03	0.01	0.2	600	3.4	58
Apple	0.2	13.4	0.5	0.3	10	14	0.660	0.000	—	—	0	1	1.0	59
Apricot Fresh	1.0	11.6	0.3	0.7	20	25	2.2	2.160	0.04	0.13	0.6	6	1.1	53
Banana	1.2	27.2	0.3	0.8	17	36	0.36	0.078	0.05	0.08	0.5	7	0.4	116
Bael	1.8	31.8	0.3	1.7	85	50	0.6	0.055	0.13	0.03	1.1	8	2.9	137
Black Berry	1.3	6.7	0.5	0.5	30	20	4.3	0.007	—	—	2.0	9	3.8	37
Cherry	1.1	13.8	0.5	0.8	24	25	0.57	0.000	0.08	0.08	0.3	7	0.4	64
Custard Apple	1.6	23.5	0.4	0.9	17	47	4.31	0.000	0.07	0.17	1.3	37	3.1	104
Dates	1.2	33.8	0.4	1.7	22	38	0.96	—	—	—	—	—	3.7	144
Phalsa	1.3	14.7	0.9	1.1	129	39	3.1	0.419	—	—	0.3	22	1.2	72
Fig	1.3	7.6	0.2	0.6	80	30	1.0	0.162	0.06	0.05	0.6	5	2.2	37
Grapes (Black or Blue)	0.6	13.1	0.4	0.9	20	23	0.5	0.003	0.04	0.03	0.2	1	2.8	58
Grapes (Pale Green)	0.5	16.5	0.3	0.6	20	30	0.52	0.000	—	—	0	1	2.9	71
Guava	0.9	11.2	0.3	0.7	10	28	0.27	0.000	0.03	0.03	0.4	212	5.2	51
Lemon	1.0	11.1	0.9	0.3	70	10	0.26	0.000	0.02	0.01	0.1	39	1.7	57

Food Items	Protein gm	Carbohydrate gm	Fat gm	Minerals gm	Calcium mg.	Phosphorus mg.	Iron mg.	Vitamin-A mg.	Vitamin-B-1 mg.	Vitamin-B-2 mg.	Vitamin-B-4 mg.	Vitamin-C mg.	Fibre gm	Energy K.Cal
	1	2	3	4	5	6	7	8	9	10	11	12	13	14
Lichi	1.1	13.6	0.2	0.5	10	35	0.7	0.000	0.02	0.06	0.4	31	0.5	61
Loquat	0.6	9.6	0.3	0.5	30	20	1.3	0.559	–	–	0	0	0.8	43
Mango	0.6	16.9	0.4	0.4	14	16	1.3	2.743	0.08	0.09	0.9	16	0.7	74
Mul Berry	1.1	10.3	0.4	0.6	70	30	2.3	0.057	0.04	0.13	0.5	12	1.1	49
Musk Melon	0.3	3.5	0.2	0.4	32	14	1.4	0.169	0.11	0.08	0.3	26	0.4	17
Orange	0.7	10.9	0.2	0.3	26	20	0.32	1.104	–	–	–	30	0.3	48
Papaya	0.6	7.2	0.1	0.5	17	13	0.5	0.666	0.04	0.25	0.2	57	0.8	32
Peach	1.2	10.5	0.3	0.8	15	41	2.4	0.000	0.02	0.03	0.5	6	1.2	50
Pear	0.6	11.9	0.2	0.3	8	15	0.5	0.028	0.06	0.03	0.2	0	1.0	52
Pine Apple	0.4	10.8	0.1	0.4	20	9	2.42	0.018	0.20	0.12	0.1	39	0.5	46
Plum (Prune)	0.7	11.1	0.5	0.4	10	12	0.6	0.166	0.04	0.1	0.3	5	0.4	52
Pomegranate	1.6	14.5	0.1	0.7	10	70	1.79	0.000	0.06	0.10	0.3	16	5.1	65
Rasp Berry	1.0	11.7	0.6	0.9	40	110	2.3	1.248	–	–	0.8	30	1.0	56

	1	2	3	4	5	6	7	8	9	10	11	12	13	14
Sapota	0.7	21.4	1.1	0.5	28	27	1.25	0.097	0.02	0.03	0.2	6	2.6	98
Strawberry	0.7	9.8	0.2	0.4	30	30	1.8	0.018	0.03	0.02	0.2	52	1.1	44
Sweet Lemon	0.7	7.3	0.3	0.5	30	20	0.7	0.000	–	0.04	0	45	0.7	35
Water Chest Nut	4.7	23.3	0.3	1.1	20	150	1.35	0.012	0.05	0.07	0.6	9	0.6	115
Water Melon	0.2	3.3	0.2	0.3	11	12	7.9	0.000	0.02	0.04	0.1	1	0.2	16

Leafy Vegetables

	1	2	3	4	5	6	7	8	9	10	11	12	13	14
Agathi (Agasti)	8.4	11.8	1.4	3.1	1130	80	3.9	5.400	0.21	0.09	1.2	169	2.2	93
Amaranth Leaves	4.0	6.1	0.5	2.7	397	83	3.49	5.520	0.03	0.30	1.2	99	1.0	45
Ambat Chuka	1.6	1.4	0.3	0.9	63	17	0.75	3.660	0.03	0.06	0.2	12	0.6	15
Bathua	3.7	2.9	0.4	2.6	150	80	4.2	1.740	0.01	0.14	0.6	35	0.8	30
Beet Leaves	3.4	6.5	0.8	2.2	380	30	16.2	5.862	0.26	0.56	3.3	70	0.7	46
Bengal Gram Leaves	7.0	14.1	1.4	2.1	340	120	23.8	0.978	0.09	0.10	0.6	61	2.0	97
Betal Leaves	3.1	6.1	0.8	2.3	230	40	10.6	5.760	0.07	0.03	0.7	5	2.3	44
Broad Bean Leaves	5.6	11.5	0.3	1.3	111	149	–	–	–	–	–	–	3.7	71

Food Items	Protein gm	Carbohydrate gm	Fat gm	Minerals gm	Calcium mg.	Phosphorus mg.	Iron mg.	Vitamin-A mg.	Vitamin-B-1 mg.	Vitamin-B-2 mg.	Vitamin-B-4 mg.	Vitamin-C mg.	Fibre gm	Energy K.Cal
	1	2	3	4	5	6	7	8	9	10	11	12	13	14
Cabbage	1.8	4.6	0.1	0.6	39	44	0.8	0.120	0.06	0.09	0.4	124	1.0	27
Carrot Leaves	5.1	13.1	0.5	2.8	340	110	8.8	5.700	0.04	0.37	2.1	79	1.9	77
Cauliflower Green	5.9	7.6	1.3	3.2	626	107	40.0	—	—	—	—	—	2.0	66
Celery Leaves	6.3	1.6	0.6	2.1	230	140	6.3	3.990	0	0.11	1.2	62	1.4	37
Colocasia Leaves	3.9	6.8	1.5	2.2	227	82	10.0	10.278	0.22	0.26	1.1	12	2.9	56
Coriander Leaves	3.3	6.3	0.6	2.3	184	71	1.42	6.918	0.05	0.06	0.8	135	1.2	44
Curry Leaves	6.1	18.7	1.0	4.0	830	57	0.93	7.560	0.08	0.21	2.3	4	6.4	108
Drum Stick Leaves	6.7	12.5	1.7	2.3	440	70	0.85	6.780	0.06	0.05	0.8	220	0.9	92
Fenu Greek Leaves	4.4	6.0	0.9	1.5	395	51	1.93	2.340	0.04	0.31	0.8	52	1.1	49

Minerals, Vitamins, Fibre and Energy Found in Different Kinds... 199

	1	2	3	4	5	6	7	8	9	10	11	12	13	14
Ipomoea	2.9	3.1	0.4	2.1	110	46	3.9	1.980	0.05	0.13	0.6	37	1.2	28
Knolkhol Leaves	3.5	6.4	0.4	1.2	740	50	13.3	4.146	0.25	–	3	157	1.8	43
Lettuce Leaves	2.1	2.5	0.3	1.2	50	28	2.4	0.990	0.09	0.13	0.50	10	0.5	21
Mint	4.8	5.8	0.6	1.9	200	62	15.6	1.620	0.05	0.26	1.0	27	2.0	48
Mustard Leaves	4.0	3.2	0.6	1.6	155	26	16.3	2.622	0.03	–	–	33	0.8	34
Neem Leaves Mature	7.1	22.9	1.0	3.4	510	80	17.1	1.998	0.04	0	1.4	218	6.2	129
Neem Leaves Tender	11.6	21.2	3.0	2.6	130	190	25.3	2.760	0.06	0	1.5	104	2.2	158
Parsley Leaves	5.9	13.5	1.0	3.2	390	175	17.9	1.920	0.04	0.18	0.5	281	1.8	87
Radish Leaves	3.8	2.4	0.4	1.6	265	59	0.09	5.295	0.18	0.47	0.8	81	1.0	28
Safflower Leaves	2.5	4.5	0.6	1.3	185	35	5.7	3.540	0.04	0.10	0	15	–	33
Spinach	2.0	2.9	0.7	1.7	73	21	1.14	5.580	0.03	0.26	0.5	28	0.6	26
Tamarind Leaves	5.8	18.2	2.1	1.5	101	140	0.30	0.250	0.24	0.17	4.1	3	1.9	115
Turnip Leaves	4.0	9.4	1.5	2.2	710	60	28.4	9.396	0.31	0.57	5.4	180	1.0	67
Water Cress Leaves	2.9	4.9	0.2	2.2	290	140	4.6	2.803	0.12	0.38	0.8	13	0.6	33

Dry Fruit/Nuts/Seeds

Food Items	Protein gm 1	Carbohydrate gm 2	Fat gm 3	Minerals gm 4	Calcium mg. 5	Phosphorus mg. 6	Iron mg. 7	Vitamin-A mg. 8	Vitamin-B-1 mg. 9	Vitamin-B-2 mg. 10	Vitamin-B-4 mg. 11	Vitamin-C mg. 12	Fibre gm 13	Energy K.Cal 14
Almond	20.8	10.5	58.9	2.9	230	490	5.09	0.000	0.24	0.57	4.4	0	1.7	655
Amaranth Seeds	14.7	60.7	1.0	3.1	510	397	11.0	–	0.07	0.21	0.5	1	9.6	319
Apricot Dry	1.6	73.4	0.7	2.8	110	70	4.6	0.058	0.22	–	2.3	2	2.1	306
Black Raisin	2.7	75.2	0.5	2.2	130	110	8.5	0.021	0.03	0.14	0.4	1	1.0	316
Cashew Nut	21.2	22.3	46.9	2.4	50	450	5.81	0.060	0.63	0.19	1.2	0	1.3	596
Coconut Dry	6.8	18.4	62.3	1.6	400	210	7.8	0.000	0.08	0.01	3.0	7	6.6	662
Coconut Fresh	4.5	13.0	41.6	1.0	10	240	1.7	0.000	0.05	0.10	0.8	1	3.6	444
Dates Dry	2.5	75.8	0.4	2.1	120	50	7.3	0.026	0.01	0.02	0.9	3	3.9	317
Groundnut	25.3	26.1	40.1	2.4	90	350	2.5	0.037	0.90	0.13	19.9	0	3.1	567

	1	2	3	4	5	6	7	8	9	10	11	12	13	14
Linseed	20.3	28.9	37.1	2.4	170	370	2.7	0.030	0.23	0.07	1.0	0	4.8	530
Melon Seeds	30.6	4.4	50.1	4.2	660	1040	17.3	–	0.13	0.20	1.3	–	0.3	607
Nigar Seeds	23.9	17.1	39.0	4.9	300	224	56.7	–	0.07	0.97	8.4	0	10.9	515
Pine Fruits	13.9	29.0	49.3	2.8	91	494	3.6	–	0.32	0.30	3.6	0	1.0	615
Pistachio Nuts	19.8	16.2	53.5	2.8	140	430	7.7	0.144	0.67	0.28	2.3	–	2.1	626
Poppy Seeds	21.7	36.8	19.3	9.9	1584	432	–	–	–	–	–	–	8.0	408
Pumpkin Seeds	24.3	15.6	47.2	4.7	50	830	5.5	0.038	0.33	0.16	3.1	1	0.2	584
Raisin	1.8	74.6	0.3	2.0	87	80	7.7	.0024	0.07	0.19	0.7	1	1.1	308
Sesame	18.3	25.0	43.3	5.2	1450	570	9.3	0.060	1.01	0.34	4.4	0	2.9	563
Sunflower Seeds	19.8	17.9	52.1	3.7	280	670	5.0	0.000	0.86	0.20	4.5	1	1.0	620
Wal Nut	15.6	11.0	64.5	1.8	100	380	2.64	0.006	0.45	0.40	1.0	0	2.6	687
Water Chest Nut (Dry)	13.4	68.9	0.8	3.1	70	440	2.4	–	–	–	–	–	–	330
Water Melon Seeds	34.1	4.5	52.6	3.7	100	937	7.4	–	0.13	0.20	1.3	–	0.8	628

Milk and Milk Products

Food Items	Protein gm	Carbohydrate gm	Fat gm	Minerals gm	Calcium mg.	Phosphorus mg.	Iron mg.	Vitamin-A mg.	Vitamin-B-1 mg.	Vitamin-B-2 mg.	Vitamin-B-4 mg.	Vitamin-C mg.	Fibre gm	Energy K.Cal
	1	2	3	4	5	6	7	8	9	10	11	12	13	14
Butter	—	—	81.0	2.5	—	—	—	0.960	—	—	—	—	—	729
Cheese	24.1	6.3	25.1	4.2	790	520	2.1	0.082	—	—	—	—	—	348
Cooking Oil-Groundnut, Mustard, Coconut, Sesame	—	—	100.0	—	—	—	—	—	—	—	—	—	—	900
Curd (Yoghurt)	3.1	3.0	4.0	0.8	149	93	0.2	0.031	0.05	0.16	0.1	1	—	60
Ghee-Buffalo	—	—	100	—	—	—	—	0.270	—	—	—	—	—	900
Ghee-Cow	—	—	100	—	—	—	—	0.600	—	—	—	—	—	900
Human Milk	1.1	7.4	3.4	0.1	28	11	—	0.041	0.02	0.02	—	3	—	65
Hydrogenated Oil-Refined	—	—	100	—	—	—	—	0.750	—	—	—	—	—	900